THE CAMPUS GUARDIAN

A Safety and Self-Protection
Handbook for Women in College and
University Settings

Simona Weber

CONTENTS

Introduction: Campus Safety and Self-Defense for Women

"I declare to you that a woman must not depend upon the protection of a man, but must be taught to protect herself, and there I take my stand."

\- Susan B. Anthony

***

In today's world, ensuring personal safety, especially on a college campus, is a priority for everyone. However, women often face unique challenges and safety concerns that require specialized knowledge and skills to navigate confidently. **"The Campus Guardian: A Safety and Self-Protection Handbook for Women in College and University Settings"** is a comprehensive handbook designed to empower women with the tools, techniques, and knowledge needed to navigate their campus and surrounding environments safely.

In recent years, the calls for greater awareness of personal safety, particularly for women on college campuses, have grown more vocal. Educational institutions are meant to be places of growth, learning, and community, yet safety concerns often plague these environments. The need for a comprehensive understanding of safety measures and self-defense strategies tailored specifically for women navigating campus life has never been more apparent.

In this book, we will address the specific safety concerns faced by women on college campuses, offering practical strategies to enhance personal safety, prevent potential threats, and build self-defense skills. By combining theoretical understanding with practical experience, you will gain the ability to recognize and evaluate possible threats, cultivate situational awareness, and apply practical self-defense tactics (when necessary) to your everyday experiences.

"The Campus Guardian: A Safety and Self-Protection Handbook for Women in College and University Settings" is not just a book about teaching physical protection techniques; it goes beyond the rudimentary self-defense techniques commonly associated with personal safety guides. While physical techniques are undoubtedly an essential component, we stress the importance of proactive measures such as risk assessment, assertive communication, and cultivating an empowerment mindset that enables college women to take charge of their safety, personal security, and well-being.

Chapter by chapter, we will explore a myriad of topics, from building a strong sense of situational awareness to comprehending the dynamics of personal safety on campuses. We will examine how to identify and neutralize possible dangers, gaining knowledge about the significance of mental readiness and emotional fortitude, in addition to physical self-defense. By the end of this book, you will have the knowledge and skills necessary to navigate your campus environment with increased resilience, self-assurance, and a heightened sense of personal security.

Understanding the Importance of Campus Safety for Women

Recognizing Potential Safety Risks and Taking Preventative Measures

"At the end of the day, the goals are simple: safety and security."

— Jodi Rell

The Reality of Campus Safety Concerns

Women are fundamentally concerned about safety in all facets of their lives, and college campuses are no different. In actuality, women's safety on college and university campuses has become a top priority, and it is a crucial subject that demands our awareness and attention. You need to be aware of the possible risks as a young lady starting this exciting new chapter in your life and take preventative action to make sure you are safe. So let's clarify the realities of campus safety concerns and provide you with the information and resources you need to face these obstacles head-on.

It is crucial to realize that no university is protected from possible dangers when it comes to campus safety. Even with their best efforts, institutions can sometimes experience crimes including theft, violence, and harassment. You can take proactive measures to safeguard yourself by accepting this fact and developing a proactive mindset. Although vibrant and educational, the university setting may often be strange and even hazardous. Women who are aware of the significance of campus safety are better equipped to take preventative action and make well-informed decisions regarding their personal protection.

To comprehend these worries, the empowerment of parents of women enrolled in colleges or universities is also extremely important. Parents can support their daughters and assist them in making decisions about their personal safety by becoming knowledgeable about issues related to campus safety.

This handbook serves as a comprehensive guide for women's safety and self-defense on college and university campuses. It addresses various topics, such as understanding the campus security infrastructure, recognizing potential risks, implementing practical safety measures, and developing self-defense skills. By following the guidance provided, you will gain the confidence needed to navigate campus life safely.

Being aware of your surroundings is one of the most important parts of campus safety. This entails being aware of your campus's layout, spotting busy, well-lit areas, and staying away from dimly lit or secluded locations, especially at night. Keeping lines of communication open with loved ones, friends, and campus security can also add an extra degree of security.

Furthermore, in an upcoming chapter, we will delve into the importance of personal safety devices such as pepper spray, personal alarms, and self-defense tools and guide you in choosing the right tools for your needs and instructions on their proper usage.

Ultimately, we aim to empower women at colleges or universities and parents of women away at colleges or universities. By understanding the reality of campus safety concerns and taking proactive measures, you can create a safer environment for yourself while pursuing your education. Remember, knowledge and preparation are powerful tools for ensuring your personal safety on campus.

***

Women's Safety and Its Effect on Academic Performance

In today's society, women's safety has become an increasingly important concern, particularly on college and university campuses. The safety and well-being of female students directly impact their academic performance and overall college experience.

Research has shown that women's focus and concentration on their academics are severely impaired when they feel intimidated or frightened. Women may struggle to completely participate in their coursework due to a persistent state of anxiety brought on by their fear of harassment, assault, or stalking. Reduced motivation, poorer grades, or even dropping out of college entirely can result from this mental anguish. To ensure their academic achievement, women must proactively address their safety concerns.

Concerns for their daughter's safety are also quite real among parents of young women who study away from home. They want to make sure that their children are safe since they are aware of the possible risks that come with living on campus. This handbook can also provide parents with the necessary tools and knowledge to support their daughters in navigating the challenges of campus safety. Through the provision of information regarding campus services, self-defense tactics, and communication strategies, parents can play an active role in promoting their daughters' safety and academic achievement.

"The Campus Guardian: A Safety and Self-Protection Handbook for Women in College and University Settings" serves as a comprehensive companion guide for women at colleges or universities, as well as their concerned parents. It not only addresses the potential dangers that women may face on campus but also offers practical solutions to mitigate these risks.

By implementing safety measures such as walking in groups, utilizing campus security services, and learning basic self-defense techniques, women can significantly reduce their vulnerability to potential threats. Additionally, the book provides valuable information on how to identify and report incidents of harassment or assault, encouraging a culture of accountability and support on campus.

Overall, the impact of women's safety on academic performance cannot be understated. When women feel safe and secure, they are more likely to thrive academically and fully engage in the college experience. We hope this handbook will serve as a vital resource for women and their parents, offering practical advice, strategies, and empowerment to ensure a safe and successful college journey.

***

The Role of Colleges and Universities in Ensuring Women's Safety

In today's modern world, where crime and safety concerns are at the forefront of everyone's minds, It is imperative to address the unique safety needs of women on college and university campuses. These educational institutions play a vital role in creating a safe and secure environment for their female students. *The Campus Guardian* handbook is intended to be an everyday, go-to resource providing practical guidance and empowering women at colleges or universities, as well as their engaged parents.

Women's safety must be given top priority in colleges and universities, both in terms of physical security and resolving the underlying problems that can lead to dangerous environments.

First and foremost, colleges and universities must establish comprehensive safety policies and protocols. This includes implementing robust security measures such as well-lit pathways, emergency call boxes, and surveillance systems. The handbook offers insights into assessing and evaluating the safety precautions already in place and encourages readers to advocate for further improvements if necessary.

Moreover, educational institutions should foster a culture of respect and consent. By promoting awareness campaigns, workshops, and training programs, colleges and universities can educate their students on the values and importance of consent, healthy relationships, and bystander intervention. Without fear of reprisals, women should feel empowered and supported to report any instances of harassment or violence.

In addition to preventive measures, colleges and universities should offer a range of support services that are specifically tailored to the needs of women. These could include access to resources for victims of sexual assault, self-defense training, and confidential counseling services. This handbook encourages readers to make use of these resources by offering a thorough list of all those that are available on campuses.

The involvement of parents of women enrolled in colleges or universities is equally important. We'll talk about their worries and stress the value of having honest conversations with their daughters. Parents who are aware of the safety precautions in place can help their daughters make wise decisions and take proactive actions to ensure their personal safety.

In conclusion, colleges and universities have a significant role in ensuring women's safety on their campuses. By implementing robust security measures, fostering a culture of respect, and providing support services, educational institutions can create an environment where women can thrive without compromising their safety. **The Campus Guardian** serves as a comprehensive guide, providing practical advice and resources for women at colleges or universities and their concerned parents. Together, we can work towards a safer future for women on campus.

"Safety and security of women and children will determine the well-being and strength of our nations."

— Rajnath Singh

3

Assessing Campus Safety Measures and Resources

Campus Security Polices, Procedures and Emergency Response Systems

Understanding Campus Security Policies and Procedures

When it comes to ensuring the safety and well-being of women on college and university campuses, understanding the campus security policies and procedures is of utmost importance. We will examine the many facets of campus security in this chapter and offer helpful guidance to assist women in navigating these policies.

Policies and procedures pertaining to campus security are implemented to safeguard students and promote a secure educational atmosphere. You may actively contribute to your own safety and the protection of people around you by becoming familiar with these rules. The particular policies and processes that are essential to know and crucial to understand are also covered in this chapter.

Firstly, we will explore emergency response protocols. Understanding the campus's emergency response system, such as the process to report incidents, contact campus security, or request emergency assistance, can save precious time in critical situations. We will also discuss the importance of having emergency contact information readily available and how to create a personal safety plan.

Next, we will discuss campus security procedures. This includes details regarding the functions and responsibilities of the security staff, as well as the existence of security cameras and emergency call boxes on campus. We'll talk about how important it is to be aware of your surroundings and how you can use safety apps or campus escort services to feel safer.

It's also critical to understand the campus policies surrounding harassment, discrimination, and sexual assault. We will give a thorough rundown of all the Title IX guidelines, methods for filing reports, and on-campus support services. Being aware of your rights and what to do in such situations is crucial for your well-being and is an empowering experience.

Finally, we will discuss ways to prevent crime. This covers advice on protecting private property, averting theft, and being secure at social gatherings and late-night pursuits. We will also stress how important it is to let friends, family, and roommates know where you are and what you are planning.

By understanding and abiding by campus security policies and procedures, women can actively contribute to creating a safe and secure campus environment. This chapter aims to equip women at college or universities, as well as their concerned parents, with the knowledge and resources necessary to navigate campus security with confidence. Empower yourself with this essential information and take control of your personal safety and well-being.

***

Evaluating Campus Lighting and Surveillance Systems

Assessing the campus lighting and monitoring systems is critical for women's safety on college and university campuses.

To create a safe environment on campus, lighting is essential. Well-lit spaces give staff and students a sense of security in addition to serving as a deterrent to would-be robbers.

You must assess the lighting on your campus:

- Are there any places, such as parking lots, quiet corners, or paths, that are dimly lit? These places may turn into potential hotspots for crime.

- Make sure you notify facilities management or campus security of any lighting issues so that the appropriate corrections can be made.

Surveillance systems, including CCTV cameras and emergency call boxes, are vital tools in enhancing campus safety.

Evaluate the coverage and visibility of the existing surveillance cameras across campus:

- Are there blind spots or areas that are not adequately monitored? Additionally, take note of where the emergency call boxes are located.

- Are they well-positioned and easy to get to in an emergency? For your safety and the safety of others, you must report any concerns you have regarding shortcomings in the surveillance system.

Consider the integration of technology in the campus security system:

- Are there any services or apps for mobile safety available to students? These apps let you instantly contact campus security or emergency services, give you real-time information on safety issues, and act as virtual escorts.

- Consider how useful and successful these tools are, then make use of them to improve your own safety.

When it comes to making sure their daughters are safe while attending colleges or universities, **parents are quite important:**

- Talk openly with your daughter about the safety precautions on campus.

- Give her the authority to report any issues to campus administrators and talk about the significance of assessing the school's lighting and security systems.

- Keep yourself updated about the institution's security procedures and have conversations with other parents to push for better security.

Improving your safety starts with assessing the lighting and security systems on your campus. You can help make your campus environment and yourself a safer place by actively participating in the evaluation process and using caution.

✳✳✳

Utilizing Emergency Call Boxes and Safe Walk Programs

One of the most important aspects of ensuring women's safety on college and university campuses is taking advantage of the various safety resources available. The safe walk programs and emergency call boxes are two key resources that every woman on campus should know about. Let's discuss these in more detail.

- **Emergency call boxes** are a vital tool for requesting assistance in an emergency and are frequently positioned strategically across campus. These boxes allow people to report any suspicious activity, threat, or emergency promptly because they have a direct line to either local law enforcement or campus security. Women should become familiar with where these call boxes are located on campus and take mental notes of their surroundings so that they can get to them promptly in case of need.

- **Safe walk initiatives** are available on many campuses in addition to emergency call boxes. These initiatives offer women a dependable means of traveling safely, particularly at night or in remote locations. Safe walk initiatives usually entail the use of volunteers or trained campus security officers who accompany people to their destinations while making sure they stay safe. These apps should be utilized by women, particularly when they are out on their own at night or in new places. It's always advisable to err on the side of caution, and having company might give you a greater sense of security.

Parents of women enrolled in colleges or universities ought to become acquainted with these resources as well. Parents can teach their daughters how to effectively use emergency call boxes and safe walk programs by having a thorough understanding of their operation. Empowering young women to take their safety seriously will come from promoting open conversation about safety concerns and the significance of using these tools.

All students, regardless of gender, should feel comfortable on campus. Women may help make the campus community a safer place for everyone by using safe walk programs and emergency call boxes. It's critical to take preventative measures for your personal safety and to always follow your gut. With the right tools and resources at hand, women can navigate their college or university experience with confidence and peace of mind.

***

Accessing Transportation Services and Campus Security Escorts

Women must have access to trustworthy security escorts and **transportation services** as they make their way through the uncharted region of college life. We will offer helpful advice on how to obtain these necessary resources, ensuring women's safety and security.

Campus security escorts are one of the best ways to improve individual safety on campus. These services are intended to give students company, especially at night or when they feel uncomfortable going places by themselves. Campus police or other security professionals with the necessary training to guarantee student safety often conduct campus security escorts.

Students are urged to familiarize themselves with the individual norms and procedures set by their different universities to gain access to campus security escorts.

Usually, the student handbook or the campus security website has this information. It is critical to be aware of the business hours, phone numbers, and any extra needs, like proof of identity or address.

Students are advised to store the campus security services' contact information in a convenient position or save it on their phones in case of an emergency or urgent necessity. This will facilitate their ability to promptly request an escort when needed. For added peace of mind, students should also let a trusted friend or family member know that they want to use the service. By doing this, they may make sure that someone is aware of their whereabouts.

Many schools provide transportation services in addition to security escorts as a safe substitute for walking alone at night. These services frequently consist of vans or shuttle buses that only go through certain zones on campus. To benefit from the convenience and increased safety of these transportation services, students should become familiar with their schedules, pick-up locations, and routes.

Women who are enrolled in colleges or universities should be encouraged by their parents to make use of these priceless resources. Parents may empower their daughters to put their personal safety first by talking to them about the value of using transportation services and security escorts. In addition, parents can help make sure their daughters always have the contact information they need on hand and that they feel free to discuss any safety concerns that may arise

Women on college and university campuses must have access to transportation services and campus security escorts. Students can safely use these tools to improve their personal safety if they are familiar with the policies and procedures set forth by their respective schools.

Parents may help their daughters by talking to them about the value of these programs and promoting their use. By working together, we can help make college campuses around the country safer places for women.

4

Developing Awareness of Your Personal Safety

Knowledge and Tools to Identify and Thwart Potential Safety Threats

"I am a Federal Air Marshal. That's the career path I chose, and for the past nineteen years, I've had a first-class ticket into the world of covert surveillance, surveillance detection, and self-defense. If I had to access all the training I've received throughout my career and pick one essential skill I could pass along to everyone I care about, It would be situational awareness."

– Gary Quesenberry

***

Identifying Potential Safety Threats on Campus

Women on college and university campuses need to be aware of any possible safety risks in their immediate environment. Through awareness of these dangers, you can take preventative action to safeguard our own security and welfare. The purpose of this chapter is to provide the information and resources you will need to recognize possible safety risks and take appropriate action.

Recognizing potential common safety hazards is one of the first steps in improving campus safety. This entails identifying locations with inadequate lighting, remote or secluded regions, or insufficient security staff. Women can plan their journeys appropriately and avoid going alone in certain places, especially at night, by being aware of these potential risk zones.

The potential for theft or assault is another security risk that should not be disregarded. Ladies should exercise caution while leaving expensive or important objects like laptops or smartphones unattended. It's also critical to exercise caution and respect for one's personal space when engaging with strangers. Following your instincts and being firm when things seem uncomfortable can help you avoid potential harm.

As previously discussed, knowing the location of emergency call boxes, emergency contact numbers, and the campus security office can be quite helpful in an emergency. With this understanding, women are more equipped to respond quickly and ask for assistance when necessary.

In addition to highlighting potential safety threats, we will also discuss the significance of self-defense training. Women can gain the knowledge and self-assurance needed to defend themselves in perilous circumstances by enrolling in self-defense training or workshops. These courses stress the value of **awareness**, **assertiveness**, and **establishing personal limits** in addition to teaching practical skills

The importance of self-defense training will be covered

in the next chapter, along with some potential safety concerns.

You can improve your personal safety and foster a secure environment by being aware of your surroundings, comprehending frequent hazards, and taking proactive measures.

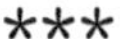

Identifying and Avoiding Dangerous Situations

Knowledge is power when it comes to personal protection. Women enrolled in colleges or universities need to be aware of the many potential risks and dangers that can occur on campus.

Trusting your instincts is the most important thing to remember. Something is probably not right if it doesn't feel right. Observe your environment and be aware of people or circumstances that give you a sense of unease or discomfort. Having faith in your instincts might help you steer clear of potentially hazardous circumstances.

A confident manner is one of the best strategies to ward off prospective attackers. Individuals who seem weak or insecure are frequently the targets of predators. You can reduce the likelihood that people will view you as an easy target by walking confidently, making eye contact, and walking with purpose.

Furthermore, become acquainted with your campus's layout and recognize locations that receive a lot of traffic and are well-lit. Follow these paths, particularly if you're out on your own at night. Steer clear of secluded regions and shortcuts, as they may make you more susceptible to danger. Try to travel with a companion if you can, or make use of the shuttle bus and escort services provided by campus security.

Technology may be a very useful tool for improving your safety as well. Make sure your smartphone is readily available and fully charged at all times. Learn how to use any emergency features or safety applications that your university may have. These tools can help you share your location with reliable contacts or provide you with rapid access to emergency services.

Setting up limits and learning to say no without feeling guilty or hesitant are also very important. Because peer pressure can occasionally result in dangerous circumstances, it's critical to put your safety and well-being first. Assemble a network of dependable pals that uphold your boundaries and promote a secure atmosphere.

Finally, make sure you let people you can trust—like friends or family—know where you are. Notify them of any changes to your plans, your extracurricular activity schedule, and your class schedule. They will be able to keep an eye on your whereabouts and check in on you as needed.

You can protect your personal safety by being proactive and avoiding dangerous situations. Remind yourself that your safety comes first and arm yourself with information and self-assurance. Maintain vigilance, believe in your gut, and take the initiative to make your campus a safe place for yourself.

***

Trust Your Gut: Listening to Your Intuition

"If you have no confidence in self, you are twice defeated in the race of life."
– Marcus Garvey

In the fast-paced and often unpredictable world of college and university campuses, women's safety should always come first. Before students set out on this exciting journey of higher education, it is critical to give them the information and resources they need to feel comfortable navigating their surroundings. A vital component of personal safety that is sometimes disregarded is the ability to use intuition, or our gut instinct's ability to warn us of impending danger or unpleasant circumstances.

Intuition is a remarkable gift that all individuals possess, but it is often dismissed or ignored due to societal conditioning or a lack of awareness. To tackle this problem head-on, we will emphasize the value of following one's intuition and offer helpful advice on how to harness this innate ability.

We encourage women to tap into their intuition as a powerful tool for personal safety. Whether it's walking alone at night, attending parties, or interacting with unfamiliar individuals, your instincts offer invaluable guidance on how to interpret and act upon your gut feelings.

There are common barriers that often prevent women from relying on their instincts, such as societal pressure or fear of being labeled as paranoid. Embrace your intuition without hesitation, emphasizing that your safety should always take precedence over societal expectations. The more you comprehend the significance of your gut feelings, the more you learn to trust them implicitly.

In the end, this subchapter is a wake-up call, encouraging women to value and believe in their instincts as an essential weapon for their own safety. By doing this, students will be able to successfully manage their time in college or university, making wise choices and staying out of potentially hazardous circumstances.

***

Practicing Situational Awareness

Developing situational awareness is one of the best strategies to improve personal safety on college and university campuses. Being aware of potential hazards and having a thorough understanding of one's surroundings can greatly lower one's likelihood of becoming a victim of crime. This section will examine the value of situational awareness and offer helpful advice on how women can hone this crucial ability.

Being fully present and observant of what is happening around you are essential components of situational awareness. It entails having the ability to evaluate your surroundings, spot possible dangers, and make wise choices to protect yourself. Women may remain ahead of the game and take proactive steps to protect themselves by adopting this mindset.

There are a few important guidelines to remember when using situational awareness. Above all, it is imperative to remain vigilant at all times. This entails staying away from distractions like using a phone excessively or turning up the volume on music. Women who maintain attention are better able to recognize cues or warning indications that may point to possible danger. Additionally, it is essential to trust your instincts. You should pay attention to your inner voice if something seems strange or unsettling. We may manage perilous situations with the help of our great intuition. It's critical to get out of a potentially dangerous situation as soon as possible.

Practicing situational awareness involves being fully conscious and perceptive of your surroundings and the people within that environment. Here are key aspects and strategies to enhance situational awareness:

Components of Situational Awareness:

- **Observation:** Pay close attention to details, including people, behaviors, and the environment.

- **Comprehension:** Understand the meaning behind observed actions or changes in the surroundings.

- **Projection:** Anticipate potential developments or changes based on gathered information.

Strategies to Improve Situational Awareness:

- **Stay Alert:** Be mentally present and avoid distractions, like using smartphones excessively, when in public spaces.

- **Scan the Environment:** Regularly scan your surroundings, looking for exits, potential threats, or unusual activities.

- **Trust Your Instincts:** Acknowledge and heed your gut feelings or intuition when sensing something is amiss.

- **Maintain Distance:** Maintain a comfortable distance from strangers or potential risks, allowing time for assessment and reaction if needed.

- **Be Mindful of Routine Changes**: Notice any alterations in familiar patterns or environments.

- **Practice Mindfulness**: Engage in mindfulness exercises to enhance awareness and focus on the present moment.

Applications in Various Settings:

- **Travel**: Stay vigilant in unfamiliar places, be cautious of pickpocketing, and familiarize yourself with emergency protocols.

- **Public Spaces**: Remain aware of surroundings in crowded areas to prevent accidents or potential threats.

- **Work Environments**: Recognize any unusual activities or changes in the workplace atmosphere that might indicate hazards or conflicts.

Benefits of Situational Awareness:

- **Personal Safety**: Helps in recognizing potential dangers and taking preemptive actions.

- **Improved Decision-Making**: Enables better decision-making by considering available information.

- **Conflict Resolution**: Allows for early detection of conflicts, facilitating timely resolution. Gary Quesenberry, Spotting Danger Before It Spots You: Build Situational Awareness to Stay Safe.

Finally, being conscious of your digital footprint is a necessary component of situational awareness development. In the current digital era, it is essential to exercise caution when sharing anything online. Don't give out personal information that can put you in danger or make you a simple target for criminals.

Situational awareness is a valuable skill that enhances personal safety, decision-making, and conflict management. Practicing vigilance and mindfulness in various settings contributes to a proactive approach in handling potential threats or challenging situations. By embracing the principles of situational awareness, women can empower themselves and take control of their personal safety on college and university campuses. The capacity to evaluate dangers, decide wisely, and react correctly is a crucial trait that can improve general well-being and safety.

5

STAY ALERT

The Colors of Situational Awareness

"Safety is something that happens between your ears, not something you hold in your hands."

– Jeff Cooper

"Situational awareness" is a concept we should be familiar with by now, but many of us don't realize that awareness alone is insufficient. "Awareness" refers to the ability to observe your surroundings and the events taking place to predict potential dangers to yourself and those in your vicinity. You have the advantage of being able to mentally and physically become ready to act should the need arise, thanks to this knowledge. Unfortunately, many people cannot take that step from being aware of a threat to taking action to address that threat because they haven't prepared their minds to take aggressive or lethal action to nullify it.

Colonel Jeff Cooper's Four-level Color Code

The late Jeff Cooper's "Color Code" has been taught by police instructors for many years. Cooper broke down situational awareness into four levels of escalating degrees of preparation for police use of deadly force. This system is a mental process, not a physical one, and should be utilized whether or not you are armed. Being alert may help you avoid a deadly threat in the first place, which is always the preferred outcome.

This method helps you move mentally from that state of mind in which you are watching out for trouble to seeing something that could be a problem and acting on it when it becomes a reality. This is called "developing your combat mindset"—that state of mind in which you are prepared to take action (whatever level of action is needed). Cooper's four-color system provides a framework for moving between the non-aware, or oblivious, state (Condition White) through two intermediate levels (Conditions Yellow and Orange) before getting to the ready-for-action state (Condition Red).

With this approach, you can move up and down this four-color continuum as the situation warrants, and you can also skip over some condition levels if the situation calls for it.

CONDITION WHITE

Condition White is a state of mind in which you have no idea what is happening around you and are ill-prepared to protect people nearby or yourself. While sleeping is the most severe example of this, many people experience this state of "unreadiness" for a large portion of the day. If there were a battle or an active shooter scenario nearby, they wouldn't notice since they are too preoccupied with their work. People in Condition White are those who are concentrating on social media interaction while using a bus or strolling down the sidewalk. They wouldn't detect anything harmful if it started to happen.

CONDITION YELLOW

In a state of relaxed alertness known as Condition Yellow, you are conscious of your surroundings and aware that something negative could happen. Not only are you gazing in front of you, but also in a 360-degree arc around yourself. But you're not doing anything about it. If you are in a location that may not be safe or if you are with people you do not know and trust, you go from Condition White to Condition Yellow. When you are in Condition Yellow, you are constantly scanning your surroundings for anything that could be dangerous or for alterations in the surroundings.

Colonel Cooper's color code is helpful in any situation where you might need to make a quick decision, not only while you're getting ready for self-defense. For instance, if a tornado notice has been issued or you feel the first tremors of a natural disaster like an earthquake, you should be in Condition Yellow.

If you see that either one is happening near you, you should immediately move into Condition Orange and think about what you need to do in your current situation and the steps you would take if you had to go to Condition Red. If the tornado moves toward you or your office building starts to shake, your trigger conditions have been tripped; you are now in Condition Red. You need to move to the storm shelter to get away from the tornado or look for a doorway to shelter under if you don't have time to get out of the building during an earthquake.

CONDITION ORANGE

Condition Orange is a state of specific alertness and awareness. As though you were in Condition Yellow, you are aware of your surroundings, but now you have recognized something or someone that might pose a hazard. You are aware that you may need to take action to counter this threat, but for the time being, you are delaying action. You also avoid developing tunnel vision and maintain an open mind by not becoming overly fixated on the potential threat that has been discovered. The last feature of Condition Orange is that you get to choose what will make you enter Condition Red by requiring an action on your part.

CONDITION RED

Condition Red indicates that you are prepared to fight or take action when necessary. When you find yourself in Condition Red, an attack or threat turns from a possible threat into a real one, and you will need to take action. It is not a reactive action but rather a planned action that you perform when a trigger condition or event materializes that you have already recognized in Condition Orange. Taking a lower degree of action, including proactively disarming the attacker, using pepper spray to blind him, knocking him out with your fists or a club, or escaping an active shooter by running out of the room, could be equivalent to shooting someone who attacks you or people nearby.

PUTTING IT ALL TOGETHER

So, to put it all together, let's think about an old Western movie. Our hero, who is never in Condition White (apart from when he is knocked out), is playing cards with a mix of friends and strangers at a table in the neighborhood saloon. He is in Condition Yellow because he is in an area that might be dangerous. Since he has his back to the wall, no one can surprise him, and he can see the entire room. He's playing cards, but when he's not gazing at his hand, he's observing the people at his table and the activities in the saloon.

He looks at the sound of the saloon doors swinging wide. He sees Black Bart and two of his cronies walk into the saloon as he glances up. He knows that Bart has been searching for him ever since he assisted the sheriff in placing Bart's younger brother in jail, which is why he is currently in Condition Orange.

While his two friends move to a table to our hero's left, Bart makes his way to the bar on his right. While concentrating on Bart, our hero keeps his eyes on the two sidekicks and surveys the room once again. Although he has recognized a few possible threats, he is only considering his options and not acting on them. He may have to use his fists, shoot someone, or decide to quietly escape out the back door to avoid any gunplay.

Having choices is a good thing. Everything hinges on what Bart and his friends decide to do. Bart sees our hero, turns around, and takes a gulp of his whiskey. A frown appears on Bart's face as his eyes narrow into slits. After discovering that he can no longer leave by the back door, our hero considers his remaining two possibilities. Right now, he's experiencing Condition Red's early phases. If the things happen that he has designated as his action triggers, he is prepared to act and use deadly force if needed.

He won't use his revolver if Bart or one of his friends approaches him without doing so, but he will definitely use the empty chair or the beer pitcher on the table as leverage if there are any physical altercations. Our hero will follow suit if one of them pulls a six-gun, eliminating Bart before turning his attention to the other two sidekicks.

The more attractive of the two sidekicks sneaks up on our hero from behind Bart, who causes a disturbance at the bar that draws his attention and enables him to be knocked unconscious by lifting the butt of his pistol.

Our hero notices the despicable attack as a shadow falls across the table. He uses his hand to find the half-empty pitcher of beer and smashes it across the sidekick's face. Then, with his Colt Peacemaker drawn, our hero turns back to Bart, whose rear is now racing out the saloon's swinging doors, followed fast by the other sidekick.

After neutralizing the detected threat, our hero returns to Condition Yellow and attempts to fill the partial flush he is holding while continuing to search the room. It's not too difficult to see oneself in a comparable scenario in a restaurant, theater, or other public setting if you give it some thought.[1]

A version of this text first appeared in the March 2017 print issue of American Survival Guide.

---

1. Larry Schwartz, American Survival Guide

6

THE IMPORTANCE OF SELF-DEFENSE TRAINING FOR WOMEN IN COLLEGE

Practical Self-Protection Principles, Techniques and Mindset

In today's society, women must be equipped with self-defense skills, particularly when attending college. College campuses, although intended to be safe spaces for learning and personal growth, unfortunately are not exempt from incidents of violence and crime. To address this pressing issue, this chapter aims to highlight the need for self-defense training, specifically tailored for women in college.

A young woman's time in college is transformative, filled with opportunities and new experiences. But it's also a period when women could be more susceptible to dangers and even more exposed to heightened risks, including sexual assault and harassment, both on and off campus. By engaging in self-defense training, women can gain the necessary skills to assert their boundaries, protect themselves, and enhance their personal safety.

***

Basic Self-Protection Principles, Techniques and Mindset

This section will cover fundamental self-defense principles, techniques, and mindset that every woman should understand. Whether you're a student at a college or university or a parent prioritizing your daughter's safety, these strategies aim to equip you with the tools needed to defend yourself in situations posing potential threats on campus. Embracing the appropriate mindset alongside practicing basic self-defense maneuvers can significantly bolster your personal security, fostering a greater sense of confidence in your capability to protect yourself.

Principles and Mindset

- **Situational Awareness:** The first line of self-defense is being aware of your surroundings. It involves being mindful of your surroundings, trusting your instincts, and recognizing potential threats. Pay attention to people and objects around you and avoid potentially dangerous situations whenever possible. Develop the habit of scanning your environment and identifying potential threats. By developing a heightened sense of awareness, you can identify potential danger and take necessary precautions. We will explore various techniques to enhance your situational awareness, such as maintaining eye contact, practicing good posture, and using peripheral vision to scan your surroundings.

- **Confidence:** Cultivating a confident mindset is crucial for self-defense. Believe in your ability to protect yourself and assert your boundaries. Confidence can deter potential attackers and give you the courage to respond effectively in tough situations.

- **Verbal Communication**: Communication skills play a vital role in self-defense. Learning to express yourself assertively and set clear boundaries can help prevent conflicts from escalating. Practice using strong, confident body language and assertive verbal commands to deter potential attackers.

- **Preparedness**: Being prepared is key to personal safety. Carry a personal safety alarm or whistle to attract attention if you feel threatened. Additionally, consider taking self-defense classes specifically tailored to your needs, such as self-defense for pregnant women or women with physical disabilities.

- **Trustworthy Relationships and Support Systems**: Surround yourself with trustworthy individuals who support your safety and well-being. Maintain open lines of communication with family, friends, and colleagues, allowing them to be aware of your whereabouts and plans.

***

Basic Self-Defense Techniques

Familiarize yourself with basic self-defense techniques that suit your physical abilities and limitations. Learn simple strikes, kicks, and escape maneuvers that can provide you with an advantage in self-defense situations. Knowing how to escape from dangerous situations is vital. Remember that the goal is to create an opportunity to escape rather than engage in a prolonged physical altercation.

- **The Palm Strike:** This move is simple yet effective. Aim for the nose or chin of your attacker and strike with the base of your palm. This technique can disorient your assailant and allow you to escape.

- **The Groin Kick:** The groin is a vulnerable area for any attacker. Use the element of surprise and deliver a swift kick to the groin. This move can incapacitate your attacker, allowing you to flee to safety.

- **The Eye Gouge:** If you find yourself in a close encounter, go for the eyes. Use your fingers to jab or poke your assailant's eyes. This move can cause extreme pain and temporarily blind your attacker, giving you a chance to escape.

- **The Elbow Strike:** When in close quarters, use your elbows as a weapon. Aim for the chin, nose, or throat of your assailant. Elbow strikes are powerful and can quickly disable your attacker.

- **The Knee Strike:** In a standing or clinching position, raise your knee and strike your assailant's groin, abdomen, or face. This move can create distance between you and your attacker, allowing you to escape.

Remember, the cornerstone of self-defense lies in being aware and ready. Stay attentive to your surroundings and trust your intuition. Moreover, consider enrolling in a women-specific self-defense program. These courses offer hands-on training, elevate confidence, and impart extra skills for effective self-protection.

For women at colleges or universities, prioritizing safety is paramount. Mastering and regularly practicing fundamental self-defense techniques will equip you to handle potentially risky situations. Encourage fellow peers to join in, raising awareness about women's safety on campus and advocating for these essential skills.

Parents, ensure that your daughters are aware of these self-defense techniques and encourage them to be proactive in their personal safety. Remind them to walk in well-lit areas, avoid isolated places, and never hesitate to reach out for help.

Remember, your safety is paramount. With knowledge, practice, and confidence, you can become the guardian of your own well-being on campus. Stay safe and empower yourself with these basic self-defense moves.

***

Self-Defense Techniques to Escape Common Holds and Grabs

In this subchapter, we will explore effective techniques to help women escape common holds and grabs, empowering them to feel safer and more confident in their daily lives on college and university campuses. Whether you are a woman attending college or a concerned parent, these techniques will provide you with valuable tools to enhance personal safety. Learning basic self-defense techniques can be crucial in times of danger. Techniques such as striking vulnerable areas like the eyes, throat, or groin can help you escape an attacker. Join self-defense classes or workshops that cater specifically to women, as they focus on techniques that work best for females. Practice these learned techniques regularly to develop muscle memory and improve your response time.

- **Escaping wrist grabs:** Wrist grabs are a common hold used by assailants to immobilize their victims. A self-defense class or workshop will demonstrate practical strategies to break free from wrist grabs, teaching you how to use leverage and strength to your advantage.

- **Countering bear hugs:** Bear hugs can be intimidating and restrict your movement. A self-defense class or workshop will teach you how to escape from this hold by utilizing effective techniques such as targeting pressure points, disrupting balance, and creating space to break free.

- **Overcoming chokeholds:** Chokeholds can be particularly dangerous and require swift action. A self-defense class or workshop will guide you through techniques to escape chokeholds, including strikes to vulnerable areas, manipulating the attacker's grip, and regaining control of the situation.

- **Defending against hair pulls:** Hair pulls can be both painful and disorienting. A self-defense class or workshop will show you how to defend against hair pulls by using proper body positioning, redirecting force, and employing effective strikes to free yourself and regain control.

- **Breaking free from arm grabs:** Arm grabs can restrict your movement and limit your ability to defend yourself. A self-defense class or workshop will demonstrate techniques to break free from arm grabs, emphasizing the importance of leverage, redirection, and maintaining your personal space.

- **Neutralizing body holds:** Body holds can leave you feeling trapped and vulnerable. A self-defense class or workshop will teach you techniques to neutralize body holds, including strikes, joint manipulation, and using the attacker's momentum against them.

Remember, these techniques are not meant to encourage confrontation but to provide you with the skills and knowledge necessary to escape potentially dangerous situations. Confidence and awareness are crucial in preventing violent encounters, but in the event of an attack, these techniques can be invaluable.

By learning and practicing these techniques regularly and maintaining a vigilant mindset, you can significantly enhance your personal safety on college and university campuses.

***

Using Pepper Spray and Other Personal Defense Devices

In today's world, personal safety has become a significant concern for women, especially those attending college or university. Consider carrying personal safety devices, such as pepper spray, a personal alarm, or a whistle. These can provide an extra layer of protection and help attract attention if you are in danger. Familiarize yourself with how to use these devices effectively and responsibly.

Pepper spray has gained popularity as a non-lethal self-defense tool, offering women a means to protect themselves from potential threats. This subchapter will address the importance of understanding local laws and regulations surrounding the possession and use of personal defense devices. By familiarizing yourself with these laws, you can confidently carry and employ pepper spray within legal boundaries.

We also explore personal defense devices, such as the use of pepper spray. Women are introduced to various other options, such as personal alarms, stun guns, and tasers, which can provide an added layer of protection. The handbook emphasizes the importance of selecting a device that aligns with one's comfort level and physical abilities.

Moreover, this subchapter delves into the psychological aspects of using personal defense devices. It highlights the importance of being mentally prepared, maintaining situational awareness, and trusting one's instincts. Women are encouraged to develop a proactive safety mindset, empowering them to respond effectively to potential dangers.

To cater to the concerns of parents, this subchapter also offers guidance to parents of women attending college or university. It provides a comprehensive overview of personal defense devices, enabling parents to understand their daughters' choices and discuss safety strategies with them.

Personal defense devices, also known as self-defense devices, are gadgets or tools designed to help individuals protect themselves in emergency situations. These devices often incorporate various technologies to provide effective defense against potential threats. Here are some of the technical aspects involved in personal defense devices:

- **Pepper Spray:** Pepper spray is a common personal defense device that uses a pressurized canister to deploy a concentrated solution of capsaicinoids, which cause irritation and temporary incapacitation. The canister typically includes a nozzle or spray mechanism to disperse the spray accurately. The concentration and spray pattern can vary depending on the specific device.

- **Stun Guns:** Stun guns deliver an electric shock to an attacker, temporarily immobilizing them. These devices usually consist of a handheld unit containing circuitry that generates high-voltage and low-amperage electrical pulses. The user applies the device directly to the attacker, allowing the electric charge to pass through their body, causing muscle contractions and pain.

- **Tasers:** Tasers are similar to stun guns but can be used from a distance. They typically employ compressed nitrogen to propel two barbed electrodes connected to conductive wires. Upon hitting the target, the electrodes deliver an electrical shock, temporarily incapacitating the attacker. Tasers often incorporate laser sights and safety mechanisms to ensure accurate and controlled deployment.

- **Personal Alarms:** Personal alarms are small, portable devices that emit a loud noise when activated. They are primarily designed to deter attackers by attracting attention and potentially scaring them off. These devices typically consist of a small electronic circuit, a battery, and a loudspeaker. Activation methods can include buttons, pull cords, or even built-in motion sensors.

- **Tactical Flashlights:** Tactical flashlights combine regular flashlight functionality with self-defense features. These flashlights often feature high-intensity LED bulbs capable of producing blinding light. Some models include strobe functions, which can disorient an attacker. Additionally, these flashlights may have a hardened bezel or a striking edge, allowing them to be used as improvised impact weapons.

- **Personal Safety Apps:** With the widespread use

of smartphones, personal safety apps have gained popularity. These apps leverage the smartphone's capabilities, such as GPS, camera, and connectivity, to provide various safety features. They may include features like emergency contacts, location sharing, loud alarms, and even automated distress messages to pre-selected contacts or authorities

- **Non-lethal Projectile Devices:** Some personal defense devices use non-lethal projectiles, such as rubber bullets, pepper balls, or bean bags, to incapacitate an attacker at a safe distance. These devices often resemble firearms and utilize compressed gas or springs to propel the projectiles. They typically incorporate aiming mechanisms, triggers, and safety features to ensure accurate and controlled deployment.

It is crucial to note that the technical aspects of personal defense devices may vary significantly depending on the design, intended use, and legal regulations in different jurisdictions. It is essential to familiarize yourself with the operation and legal implications of any personal defense device before use.

Strategies for Safeguarding Yourself During Solo Travel

When it comes to traveling alone, safety should always be a top priority. Women enrolled in college or university settings may encounter distinct challenges and potential risks, particularly when traveling alone for work, whether on or off-campus, or commuting between home and school. In this section, we will explore practical self-protection principles specifically designed to guide college women who often travel solo.

- **Awareness and preparation:** The first line of defense is being aware of your surroundings and taking precautions. Research your destination, familiarize yourself with local customs and laws, and share your travel itinerary with a trusted friend or family member. Additionally, consider taking a self-defense course before your trip to build confidence and learn essential techniques.

- **Maintain good body language:** Confidence is key. Walk with purpose, maintain good posture, and make eye contact with those around you. This sends a message that you are aware and not an easy target.

- **Plan your transportation:** When using public transportation or taxis, choose reputable companies and avoid traveling alone late at night. If possible, sit near the driver or with other passengers. Always let someone know your transportation plans and estimated arrival time.

- **Share your itinerary:** Share your travel plans with trusted contacts and keep them updated on your whereabouts.

- **Trust your instincts:** Your intuition is a powerful tool. If a situation or person makes you uncomfortable, trust your gut and remove yourself from it. Avoid isolated areas, especially at night, and always stay in well-lit and populated areas.

- **Blend in and limit exposure:** Dressing appropriately and blending in with the local culture can help you avoid drawing unnecessary attention. Research local customs and dress modestly, if necessary. Avoid wearing flashy jewelry or carrying expensive belongings that may attract thieves.

- **Keep essentials close:** Carry essentials like money, a phone, and an ID in a secure, easily accessible place.

- **Use technology wisely:** Utilize smartphone apps and devices to enhance your safety. Share your location with trusted contacts, install personal safety apps, and program emergency numbers into your phone. Additionally, consider carrying a personal safety alarm or a whistle to attract attention in case of an emergency.

- **Stay connected:** Keep your phone charged and maintain communication with family or friends.

- **Local emergency numbers:** Save local emergency contacts or embassy numbers in your phone.

- **Backup important documents:** Store digital copies of passports, IDs, and travel documents in secure cloud storage.

- **Use reliable apps:** Utilize trusted travel apps for navigation, language translation, and emergency assistance.

- **Learn and employ the basic self-defense techniques:** Being equipped with basic self-defense techniques can provide you with confidence and a sense of security. Focus on moves that require minimal strength or physical contact, such as strikes to sensitive areas, joint locks, and escapes from common grabs. Remember, self-protection is not just physical; it includes mental and emotional preparedness. Trust your instincts, be aware of your surroundings, and take proactive steps to ensure your safety while traveling alone. Solo travel offers incredible experiences but requires a proactive approach to personal safety. By planning ahead, staying vigilant, securing belongings, and maintaining communication, you can enhance your safety and enjoy your journey confidently.

✳✳✳

Understanding the Legalities of Self-Defense

When it comes to personal safety, understanding the legal aspects of self-defense holds significant importance and ensures that individuals protect themselves within the confines of the law. However, it's crucial to note that self-defense laws differ across jurisdictions, underscoring the importance of acquainting yourself with the specific laws in your region. While this section offers a general outline, consulting local legal resources is strongly advised for a comprehensive understanding.

Here are some essential aspects to consider regarding the legalities of self-defense:

Legal Definition:

- **Right to Self-Defense:** Laws generally recognize the right of individuals to defend themselves from imminent harm or threats.

- **Proportional Force:** Individuals are allowed to use reasonable and proportional force necessary to counter an immediate threat. The central tenet of self-defense revolves around the notion of proportional force. The force used in self-defense should match the level of the perceived threat. This implies using only the necessary force to halt the threat and ensure your protection

It is crucial to note that self-defense laws differ across jurisdictions, underscoring the importance of acquainting yourself with the specific laws in your region.

Elements of Self-Defense:

- **Imminent Threat:** The threat must be immediate or ongoing to justify a self-defense response.

- **Reasonable Belief:** The individual must have a reasonable belief that their safety or someone else's safety is in danger.

- **Proportional Response:** The response used for self-defense should align with the threat faced and not exceed it.

Duty to Retreat vs. Stand Your Ground:

- **Duty to Retreat:** Some jurisdictions require individuals to attempt to retreat or avoid the confrontation before resorting to self-defense.

- **Stand Your Ground:** Other jurisdictions have "stand your ground" laws, allowing individuals to defend themselves without the obligation to retreat.

It's essential to comprehend your jurisdiction's position on this issue to ensure compliance with the law.

Avoidance of Aggression:

- **Initiating Violence:** Acting aggressively or initiating force when not facing an immediate threat can lead to legal consequences.

- **Preemptive Strikes:** Preemptive strikes or use of force without a valid threat might not qualify as self-defense under the law.

It's crucial to differentiate between self-defense and aggression. Engaging in self-defense entails reacting to an imminent threat or peril. However, initiating violence or using force when not facing immediate danger does not constitute self-defense and might result in legal repercussions.

Reporting and Documentation:

- **Reporting Incidents:** It's advisable to report instances where self-defense is used to the relevant authorities

- **Documentation:** Keeping records or evidence of the incident, witnesses, and actions taken can support one's self-defense claim if legal proceedings arise.

This documentation will serve to bolster your case in the event of legal proceedings.

Varied Legal Standards:

- **Jurisdiction Differences:** Self-defense laws can vary significantly by state or country, and understanding local laws is vital.

- **Case-by-Case Basis:** Legal assessments of

self-defense claims are often evaluated on a case-by-case basis considering the circumstances.

Seek Legal Advice:

- **Consult Legal Experts**: When in doubt or facing legal inquiries, seeking advice from legal professionals knowledgeable about self-defense laws is recommended.

- **Education and Awareness**: Understanding the legal framework around self-defense empowers individuals to protect themselves effectively while staying within legal boundaries.

Grasping the legal intricacies of self-defense enables you to fortify your ability to protect yourself while ensuring adherence to the law and prioritizing your personal safety.

Whether it's understanding the legalities, learning proper techniques, or exploring different personal defense devices, this chapter aims to ensure that women and their parents are well-informed and prepared in their pursuit of safety and security. Self-protection extends beyond physical techniques; it involves cultivating a resilient mindset and embracing proactive approaches to mitigate risks. Integrating these fundamental principles and mindset into your everyday routine bolsters your personal safety, empowering you to confidently navigate your college or university campus and diverse environments.

To summarize, the importance of self-defense training for women in college is unquestionable. Acquiring the essential skills and knowledge empowers you to traverse your college years with confidence in your personal safety. This readiness allows you to assert control over your safety both within and beyond college and university campuses, guiding you throughout your life.

7

Developing Physical and Mental Fortitude

The Significance of Physical Fitness, Mental Resilience and Self-Care for Your Safety and Well-Being

"The self is not something ready-made, but something in continuous formation through choice of action."

— John Dewey

Incorporating Physical Fitness into Your Routine

Physical fitness is not only important for maintaining a healthy body but also plays a crucial role in women's safety and self-defense on college and university campuses. It's important to understand the significance of physical fitness and how to incorporate it into your daily routine.

Regular exercise has numerous benefits, including increased strength, improved cardiovascular health, enhanced mental well-being, and reduced stress levels. Engaging in physical activity can also boost self-confidence and self-esteem, which are essential attributes for personal safety. By incorporating physical fitness into your routine, you empower yourself to be more alert, agile, and capable of defending yourself if the need arises. Focus on exercises that enhance core strength and flexibility.

It is important to find activities that suit your interests and fit your schedule. Whether it's joining a sports team, attending fitness classes, or simply going for a jog, there are numerous options available on college campuses to help you stay active. The handbook provides practical tips on how to access these resources and make the most of them.

Additionally, we emphasize the importance of setting realistic goals and creating a consistent exercise routine. It provides advice on how to start slowly and gradually increase the intensity of your workouts. By taking small steps and sticking to a plan, you can ensure that physical fitness becomes a sustainable part of your lifestyle.

Furthermore, the handbook highlights the significance of self-defense training alongside physical fitness. It encourages women to enroll in self-defense classes, where they can learn crucial techniques to protect themselves in dangerous situations. These classes not only provide valuable skills but also instill a sense of empowerment and confidence.

For parents, it's important to support your daughters in incorporating physical fitness into their college routine by encouraging a healthy lifestyle, discussing the importance of fitness, and ensuring their access to appropriate facilities and resources on campus.

Incorporating physical fitness into your routine is a vital aspect of women's safety and self-protection on college and university campuses. We have provided valuable insights, practical advice, and resources to help women prioritize physical fitness and create a safer environment on campus. By taking control of your physical well-being, you can enhance your personal safety and empower yourself in all aspects of your life.

✳✳✳

Developing Mental Resilience and Confidence

In a world where personal safety is a growing concern, it is crucial for women on college and university campuses to not only possess physical self-defense skills but also develop mental resilience and confidence. The ability to navigate challenging situations, trust one's instincts, and maintain a strong sense of self is essential for women's safety and overall well-being. Let's discuss the importance of mental resilience and confidence-building techniques specifically tailored to women in higher education.

For women at colleges or universities, developing mental resilience and confidence is about equipping oneself with the tools to handle potentially dangerous situations effectively. It starts with understanding the power of mindset and the impact it can have on personal safety. By adopting a proactive and empowered mindset, women can approach their college experience with a sense of self-assurance and preparedness. Cultivating a resilient and confident mindset is crucial for women to navigate college life and all its challenges effectively. Here are some practical tips and exercises tailored to help foster resilience and confidence:

Visualization Techniques:

- **Future Self Visualization:** Close your eyes and visualize your future self as a confident, resilient person. Envision scenarios where you handle challenges with grace and poise. Feel the emotions associated with that confidence. Repeat this exercise regularly to reinforce the image.

- **Outcome Visualization:** Picture successful outcomes for situations causing stress. Visualize yourself overcoming obstacles and achieving your goals. This helps in creating a positive mental framework and prepares you for potential hurdles.

Positive Self-Talk:

- **Affirmations:** Create affirmations that resonate with you. Repeat these positive statements daily, focusing on strengths, abilities, and resilience. For example, "I am strong, capable, and worthy of success."

- **Gratitude Journaling:** Write down things you're grateful for regularly. Acknowledging positives in your life can boost confidence and resilience by shifting focus to what's going right.

Setting Personal Boundaries:

- **Identify Boundaries:** Reflect on your personal values and what makes you comfortable or uncomfortable in various situations. Define clear boundaries for yourself in relationships, work, and personal life.

- **Communicate Boundaries:** Assertively communicate your boundaries to others. Practice saying no when something doesn't align with your values or makes you uncomfortable. Remember, setting boundaries is a sign of self-respect.

Exercises for Resilience:

- **Challenge Interpretation:** When facing a setback, reframe it as a learning opportunity. Ask yourself, "What can I learn from this?" or "How can I grow stronger through this experience?"

- **Stress Management Techniques:** Incorporate stress-relieving activities like meditation, deep breathing exercises, yoga, or hobbies. These practices can build emotional resilience and improve overall well-being.

- **Reflect and Learn:** After overcoming a challenging situation, reflect on what helped you cope. Identify your strengths and strategies that were effective. Use this knowledge as a resource for future difficulties.

- **Progressive Goal Setting:** Break larger goals into smaller, manageable steps. Celebrate achievements along the way, reinforcing your confidence in your abilities.

Building resilience and confidence is an ongoing process. Consistency and self-compassion are key. Combine these exercises and techniques to create a personalized routine that suits your needs and helps you thrive in your college years. If necessary, seek support from a therapist or counselor to further explore these practices and tailor them to your specific circumstances.

Parents also play a vital role in supporting their daughters' safety and well-being while they are away at college. We acknowledge your concerns and encourage guidance on fostering mental resilience and confidence from a distance, such as proactive communication with your daughters, providing them with resources such as safety apps and emergency contacts, and encouraging participation in self-defense classes or workshops. By being a proactive advocate for your daughters' personal safety, you help to alleviate their concerns and equip them with the necessary knowledge and tools to help fortify their safety.

As a comprehensive handbook, we not only focus on physical self-defense techniques but also recognize the importance of mental resilience and confidence. By addressing the unique challenges faced by women on college and university campuses, we hope we have provided practical guidance, tips, and exercises to help you develop the necessary mental fortitude to navigate potentially unsafe situations.

***

Practicing Self-Care and Stress Management

Amid the fast-paced and demanding college or university environment, women need to prioritize their well-being and adopt proactive measures to handle stress. Our goal is to empower women on campuses by offering practical strategies for self-care and stress management, enabling them to navigate their academic journeys more effectively.

College life can be overwhelming with the pressure to excel academically, navigate social relationships, and adjust to new surroundings. It is essential to recognize the importance of self-care and its positive impact on overall mental and physical health. By incorporating self-care practices into their daily routines, women can cultivate resilience, reduce stress levels, and enhance their overall well-being.

Various self-care techniques can benefit women on college or university campuses. We have emphasized the significance of setting boundaries, managing time effectively, and prioritizing self-care activities. We encourage women to engage in activities that bring joy and relaxation, such as exercise, mindfulness, journaling, or spending time in nature.

Moreover, stress management is a critical skill for women on campuses. Some practical strategies to cope with stress effectively include deep breathing exercises, meditation, and progressive muscle relaxation that can help women reduce anxiety and promote mental clarity. Coping with stress effectively is essential, especially for women dealing with various pressures. Here are practical strategies that can significantly help in reducing anxiety and promoting mental clarity:

Deep Breathing Exercises:

Diaphragmatic Breathing (Belly Breathing):

- Sit or lie down comfortably.

- Place one hand on your belly and the other on your chest.

- Inhale deeply through your nose, feeling your belly rise. Ensure your chest remains still.

- Exhale slowly through your mouth, feeling your belly fall.

- Repeat this deep breathing pattern several times, focusing on rhythm and relaxation.

4-7-8 Breathing Technique:

- Inhale quietly through your nose for a count of 4.

- Hold your breath for a count of 7.

- Exhale forcefully through your mouth for a count of 8.

- Repeat this cycle a few times to induce relaxation.

Meditation:

Mindfulness Meditation:

- Find a quiet place and sit comfortably or lie down.

- Focus on your breath or choose a specific point of focus (like a mantra or an object).

- Allow thoughts to come and go without judgment, gently bringing your focus back to your chosen point of concentration.

- Practice for a few minutes daily, gradually increasing the duration.

Progressive Muscle Relaxation (PMR):

Guided PMR:

- Find a quiet, comfortable space and close your eyes.

- Starting from your toes, systematically tense and then relax each muscle group in your body.

- Focus on the contrast between tension and relaxation.

- Move upward, tensing and relaxing each muscle group, including legs, abdomen, arms, neck, and facial muscles.

Additional Tips for Stress Management:

- **Regular Exercise:** Engage in physical activity as it releases endorphins, which can reduce stress and improve mood.

- **Healthy Lifestyle:** Prioritize a balanced diet, adequate sleep, and hydration to support your body in handling stress.

- **Setting Boundaries:** Learn to say no when necessary, and don't overcommit. Respect your limitations and prioritize self-care.

- **Seek Support:** Talk to friends, family, or a counselor when feeling overwhelmed. Having a support system is crucial.

These techniques and practices can be incorporated into daily routines to manage stress effectively. Experiment with different methods and find what works best for you. Consistency is key, so practice regularly to experience their full benefits in reducing anxiety and enhancing mental clarity.

We acknowledge the unique challenges faced by women in college or university environments and stress the significance of building a strong support network, including friends, family, and campus resources. We also encourage women to take advantage of counseling services or support groups available on campus.

We acknowledge the comprehensive importance of personal well-being and encourage women to prioritize both their mental and physical health while maneuvering through college life.

8

ENHANCING COMMUNICATION SKILLS AND ASSERTIVENESS

Empowering Your Voice

Developing Assertive Techniques for Establishing Boundaries

In this chapter, we explore the significance of assertiveness skills concerning women's safety and self-defense in college and university environments. Our focus will be on practical strategies that aid women in effectively setting and upholding their personal boundaries.

As a woman in college or university, it's vital to understand that establishing boundaries is both your entitlement and your duty. By articulating your limits clearly, you empower yourself and convey your expectations clearly to others. Parents of women attending colleges or universities can also benefit from grasping these skills to assist their daughters in safely navigating campus life.

First and foremost, it's crucial to cultivate self-awareness and comprehend your values, necessities, and comfort thresholds. Being in tune with yourself will help you recognize situations that might challenge your boundaries. Trust your instincts and heed your inner feelings when something seems amiss. Your intuition serves as a potent asset in evaluating potential risks.

Once you are aware of your boundaries, it becomes vital to assertively convey them to others. Practice employing "I" statements to directly and courteously express your needs and limits. For instance, phrases like "I feel uncomfortable with that" or "I need some space right now" effectively communicate your boundaries without assigning blame or attacking others. Moreover, maintaining eye contact and speaking in a composed yet firm tone can amplify your assertiveness.

However, it's crucial to recognize that establishing boundaries might encounter resistance or opposition from others. In such instances, it's essential to stand firm and uphold your assertiveness. Bear in mind, your safety and well-being are of utmost importance, and you hold the right to prioritize them.

Moreover, establishing and sustaining a support network plays a crucial role in effectively upholding your boundaries. Surround yourself with friends, family, or support groups who honor and bolster your limits. Their support and empathy will furnish you with the assurance and reinforcement required to remain steadfast in your boundaries.

Finally, it's crucial to periodically review and adjust your boundaries as necessary. College and university experiences are fluid, and circumstances may evolve. Maintaining flexibility and modifying your boundaries accordingly will assist you in navigating new challenges and ensuring your continued safety.

To sum up, mastering assertiveness skills is pivotal for establishing and upholding boundaries, and promoting women's safety and self-defense across college and university campuses. Through cultivating self-awareness, proficiently expressing your limits, maintaining resilience, and seeking support, you empower yourself to foster a safe and secure environment. Always remember that your boundaries hold significance, and you possess the right to safeguard yourself and your well-being.

***

Communicating Clearly and Confidently in Unsafe Situations

When it comes to personal safety, effective communication can play a crucial role in diffusing potentially dangerous situations. In this subchapter, we will explore the importance of clear and confident communication, and offering practical advice tailored for women at college and university campuses.

- **The Power of Assertive Communication**: Assertiveness is key when it comes to personal safety. By expressing yourself confidently and clearly, you can establish boundaries and deter potential threats. Some techniques to enhance your assertiveness skills are maintaining strong body language, using a firm and clear voice, and practicing effective eye contact.

- **Verbal De-Escalation Strategies**: In unsafe situations, knowing how to de-escalate conflicts through verbal communication can be a valuable tool. Effective de-escalation strategies are invaluable in defusing tense situations and mitigating the risk of violence. Here are examples of techniques that can be highly effective:

Active Listening:

Active listening involves fully concentrating, understanding, responding, and remembering what is being said. It shows respect and understanding, which can defuse tension. Key elements include:

- **Attentive Posture:** Maintain an open and non-threatening body language to show interest and engagement.

- **Reflective Responses:** Reflect back on what the other person is saying to ensure understanding.

- **Clarifying Questions:** Ask questions to gain more insight and show genuine interest in their perspective.

Empathy:

Empathy is the ability to understand and share the feelings of another person. It helps in creating a connection and reducing tension by acknowledging the other person's emotions. Techniques include:

- **Acknowledging Feelings:** Validate the other person's emotions by acknowledging their feelings. For example, "I understand you're feeling upset."

- **Showing Understanding:** Communicate understanding by reflecting on their situation. This shows that you're listening and empathizing with their perspective.

Use of "I" Statements:

- "I" statements focus on expressing your feelings, thoughts, and opinions without attributing blame. They can prevent defensiveness and aggression by keeping the conversation non-confrontational. For example:

- Instead of saying, "You're making me angry," say,

"I feel upset when this happens."

- Replace "You're wrong" with "I see things differently."

Additional Tips:

- **Remain Calm:** Keep your emotions in check to prevent escalation.

- **Respect Personal Space:** Maintain a respectful physical distance to avoid making the situation more intense.

- **Avoid Aggressive Body Language:** Refrain from gestures or expressions that could be interpreted as aggressive.

Practice and Application:

- Role-play scenarios to practice these de-escalation techniques.

- In real-life situations, use these strategies calmly and sincerely.

These de-escalation techniques are crucial in diffusing conflicts, promoting understanding, and preventing potentially violent situations from escalating. They empower individuals to communicate effectively and resolve issues in a non-confrontational manner, promoting safety and harmony in various environments.

Non-Verbal Communication Cues:

Non-verbal cues can speak volumes in dangerous situations, often influencing the behavior of those around you. Understanding the significance of body language, facial expressions, and posture is crucial, as they convey confidence and can serve as deterrents to potential attackers. Here's why being mindful of these non-verbal cues is important:

Confident Body Language:

- **Positive Posture:** Standing tall with an upright posture communicates confidence and assertiveness. It projects a sense of self-assurance that may discourage potential threats.

- **Maintaining Eye Contact:** Sustaining appropriate eye contact portrays confidence and attentiveness. It indicates that you're aware of your surroundings and can discourage individuals seeking vulnerability.

Assertive Facial Expressions:

- **Neutral and Composed:** Keep your facial expressions neutral and composed. Avoid showing fear or anxiety, as it might signal vulnerability.

- **Confidence in Expressions:** Projecting calmness and confidence through facial expressions can act as a deterrent. It can communicate that you're alert and capable of handling situations.

Body Language Awareness:

- **Open and Relaxed Gestures:** Avoid crossing arms or making defensive gestures, as these can convey vulnerability. Open and relaxed gestures can communicate confidence and openness.

- **Awareness of Personal Space:** Be mindful of your personal space. Standing too close or too far from others may send unintended signals. Maintain a comfortable distance to assert boundaries.

Importance in Deterrence:

Being conscious of your body language, facial expressions, and posture isn't just about self-presentation. It's a powerful tool in deterring potential attackers or threats:

- **Projecting Confidence:** Confident body language may dissuade potential attackers, as it suggests you're aware, assertive, and less likely to be an easy target.

- **Signaling Awareness:** Being attentive to your surroundings with confident body language signals that you're alert and prepared, making you less susceptible to attacks.

- **Setting Boundaries:** Assertive body language can deter individuals who might perceive passivity or vulnerability as an opportunity.

Practice and Awareness:

- Practice confident body language and assertive postures in everyday situations to make it a habit.

- Regularly assess your non-verbal cues to ensure they convey confidence and alertness.

Utilizing Technology for Safety:

In today's digital age, technology can be a powerful ally in enhancing personal safety. Leveraging technology through smartphone apps, wearable devices, and safety features can be invaluable in discreetly and swiftly communicating during emergencies. Here are some options:

Smartphone Apps:

- **Safety Apps:** Numerous safety apps are available that offer features like sending SOS alerts to emergency contacts, sharing real-time location, and activating distress signals discreetly.

- **Personal Safety Networks:** Apps that establish a network with trusted contacts, allowing them to track your location, receive check-in notifications, and send alerts in emergencies.

- **Emergency Call Apps:** Some apps simplify the emergency call process by connecting you directly to the local emergency services or providing essential information to responders.

Wearable Devices:

- **Safety Wearables:** Devices like smartwatches or discreet panic buttons can trigger emergency alerts when activated. They often sync with smartphones to send distress signals or share location details.

- **Smart Jewelry:** Wearables in the form of jewelry (rings, bracelets) equipped with safety features like discreetly calling for help, sending distress signals, or recording audio/video.

Safety Features on Smartphones:

- **Emergency SOS Feature:** Most smartphones have built-in emergency features that allow users to quickly call emergency services by pressing specific buttons or using voice commands.

- **Location Sharing:** Smartphones often have location-sharing functionalities that can be used to share real-time whereabouts with trusted contacts or emergency services.

- **Voice-Activated Assistance:** Voice-activated assistants on smartphones can be programmed to call emergency services or send SOS messages by voice commands.

Importance and Tips:

- **Pre-Set Contacts:** Configure these apps or devices with trusted emergency contacts.

- **Test and Familiarize:** Ensure you are familiar with how these apps or devices work by conducting practice sessions.

- **Charging and Accessibility:** Keep devices charged and easily accessible, especially in situations where quick access might be crucial.

Considerations:

- **Privacy and Permissions:** Be aware of the permissions granted to these apps and devices, especially regarding location tracking and data sharing.

- **Network Coverage:** Ensure that these tools work in areas with adequate network coverage or have offline functionalities.

- **Preparing for Difficult Conversations:** Sometimes, assertive communication may be required in difficult conversations with acquaintances, friends, or even authority figures. Navigating conversations where you want to ensure your concerns are heard and addressed appropriately requires thoughtful preparation and effective communication strategies. Here's guidance on preparing for and navigating such discussions:

Clarify Your Concerns:

- **Identify Specific Concerns:** Pinpoint the exact issues or situations you want to address. Be clear about what's bothering you or what needs to change.

- **Consider Desired Outcomes:** Determine what you hope to achieve from the conversation. Whether it's seeking understanding, solutions, or a behavior change, having clear goals is essential.

Plan and Prepare:

- **Choose the Right Time and Place:** Opt for a suitable environment that is conducive to an open and respectful conversation. Ensure privacy and minimize distractions.

- **Organize Your Thoughts:** Structure your points logically to express yourself clearly and coherently. Consider writing down key points to avoid forgetting important details.

Effective Communication:

- **Active Listening:** Be attentive to the other person's perspective. Listen actively to understand their viewpoint without interrupting.

- **Use "I" Statements:** Frame your concerns using "I" statements to express your feelings and experiences without attributing blame. For instance, say, "I feel concerned when..." rather than "You always..."

Stay Calm and Respectful:

- **Remain Calm:** Control your emotions to keep the conversation constructive. Take deep breaths or pause if emotions escalate.

- **Respectful Tone and Body Language:** Maintain a respectful tone and open body language to foster a non-confrontational atmosphere.

Be Open to Solutions:

- **Collaborative Approach:** Encourage a collaborative discussion by being open to solutions and alternatives. Work together toward resolving the concerns.

- **Seek Understanding:** Encourage the other person to share their perspective. This promotes mutual understanding and helps find common ground.

Follow-Up and Closure:

- **Confirm Understanding:** Ensure both parties understand each other's viewpoints and agreed-upon actions.

- **Follow-Up Plans:** If needed, outline follow-up steps or actions to address the concerns discussed.

Additional Tips:

- **Practice Empathy:** Put yourself in the other person's shoes to better understand their perspective.

- **Set Boundaries:** Clearly articulate your boundaries and what you consider acceptable.

- **Seek Support:** If necessary, seek guidance from a trusted friend or counselor to prepare for the conversation.

Effective preparation, clear communication, maintaining composure, and being open to resolution are key aspects of preparing for and navigating conversations where your concerns need to be heard and addressed appropriately. By employing these strategies, you can foster productive discussions and increase the likelihood of achieving a positive outcome.

- **Building a Support Network:** Having a strong support network is essential for personal safety. It is important to build connections with trusted friends, family, and campus resources so you can effectively communicate your concerns to loved ones and seek their support.

Through adept and assured communication, women on college and university campuses can equip themselves to maneuver through potentially risky situations. Whether employing assertive body language, practicing de-escalation methods, or leveraging technology, mastering effective communication skills substantially bolsters personal safety. Always keep in mind that your safety is paramount, and communication stands as a potent asset in your self-defense toolkit.

***

Reporting Incidents and Seeking Support from Campus Authorities

Within the vibrant atmosphere of college and university campuses, prioritizing women's safety stands as a pivotal concern. Women must comprehend the resources accessible to them and understand the process of seeking aid from campus authorities during incidents. This section strives to provide women at colleges or universities, along with parents of female students attending these institutions, with the necessary knowledge and abilities to navigate such circumstances.

In moments of crisis, maintaining composure and evaluating the situation is the initial step. It's crucial to recognize that you're not alone, and support is readily available. Reporting incidents to campus authorities plays a pivotal role in fostering a safer environment for everyone. Begin by identifying suitable channels for reporting incidents, such as the campus police, security office, or women's center. These resources are tailored to address diverse situations, encompassing physical assault, harassment, stalking, and various forms of misconduct.

It's essential to promptly and comprehensively document all incidents. Maintain a record detailing dates, times, locations, incident descriptions, and any witnesses present. This documentation serves as crucial evidence, aiding authorities in taking suitable actions. Moreover, consider reaching out to witnesses and encouraging them to offer statements or support for your case if they feel comfortable doing so.

When reporting an incident, be ready to recount your experience and offer as much detail as you can. Remember, these authorities exist to offer support and safeguard you. Share your worries, apprehensions, and any pertinent information you believe is important. They'll assist you throughout the process, elucidate your rights, and offer information regarding accessible resources, including counseling services, legal aid, or support groups.

Moreover, maintaining open communication with campus authorities during the investigation is critical. Consistently check on the status of your case and offer any new information that emerges. Always bear in mind, your safety and well-being hold utmost importance, and advocating for yourself is crucial.

In this subchapter, we have highlighted the importance of reporting incidents and seeking support from campus authorities. Remember, you are not alone, and together, we can create a community that prioritizes women's safety and well-being.

9

NAVIGATING SAFELY IN SOCIAL AND PARTY ENVIRONMENTS

Making Informed Decisions and Prioritizing Safety

Understanding the Risks of Alcohol and Drug Use

In this handbook, we must address the risks associated with alcohol and drug use. This subchapter aims to educate women at colleges or universities about the potential dangers and consequences that can arise from these substances. By providing this information, we hope to empower college women to make informed decisions and prioritize their safety.

College and university campuses are frequently associated with social gatherings and events where alcohol and drug consumption might be common. While acknowledging that responsible drinking is part of the college experience for some, it's equally crucial to comprehend the associated risks. Excessive alcohol intake can hinder judgment, coordination, and decision-making capabilities, heightening vulnerability to hazardous situations. Women, especially, might encounter amplified risks like sexual assault or harassment when affected by alcohol.

Both illicit and prescription drugs carry substantial risks. Consumption of substances like marijuana, cocaine, or opioids can impede cognitive function, distort perception, and heighten the chances of participating in perilous behavior. Furthermore, misusing prescription drugs like stimulants or painkillers can lead to severe consequences for both physical and mental health.

Women should understand potential hazards and adopt proactive measures to reduce risks. Here are some practical steps to consider:

- **Educating yourself**: Familiarize yourself with the impacts of alcohol and different drugs, encompassing both their immediate and lasting effects. Understanding these risks can aid in making well-informed choices.

- **Setting boundaries**: Establish personal limits regarding alcohol and drug use. It's essential to know your limits and respect them to maintain control over your actions and safety.

- **Practicing responsible drinking**: If you choose to drink, do so in moderation. Pace yourself, alternate alcoholic beverages with non-alcoholic ones, and always stay hydrated. Surround yourself with trusted friends who can help look out for each other's well-being.

- **Being mindful of your surroundings**: When attending parties or social events, be aware of your environment. Stay in well-lit areas, avoid isolated spaces, and trust your instincts if you feel uncomfortable.

- **Utilizing campus resources**: Familiarize yourself with the support services available on campus. Many universities provide counseling, helplines, or student organizations dedicated to substance abuse prevention and support.

By understanding the risks associated with alcohol and

drug use, women can make informed choices that prioritize their safety and well-being. We emphasize the importance of being proactive, setting boundaries, and seeking support when needed. Ultimately, every woman deserves to feel safe and empowered as they navigate their college experience.

***

Strategies for Safe Socializing and Partying

As a woman attending college or university, it is crucial to prioritize your safety while socializing and partying. Let's discuss essential strategies to navigate these environments confidently and minimize potential risks.

- **Stay Alert and Trust Your Intuition**: The most effective way to stay safe is by being aware of your surroundings and trusting your instincts. If a situation feels uncomfortable or unsafe, remove yourself from it immediately.

- **Buddy System**: Always go out with a trusted friend or group of friends. Look out for each other and establish a code word or signal to communicate when one of you feels uncomfortable or needs assistance.

- **Plan Ahead**: Before attending a social event or party, inform a trusted friend or family member about your plans, including the location, duration, and who you will be with. Set a time to check in with them during the event.

- **Be Mindful of Alcohol Consumption**: Limit your alcohol intake and know your limits. Excessive drinking can impair your judgment and increase vulnerability. Watch your drink at all times to prevent tampering.

- **Utilize Campus Resources:** Familiarize yourself with campus safety resources, such as a campus escort service, emergency call boxes, or self-defense classes. Take advantage of these resources to enhance your personal safety.

- **Plan Your Transportation:** Avoid walking alone at night, especially in unfamiliar or poorly lit areas. Utilize campus shuttles, and rideshare services, or arrange for a trusted friend to accompany you.

- **Trustworthy Social Connections:** Be cautious when making new friends or accepting invitations from unfamiliar individuals. Get to know people gradually and trust your instincts when deciding who to spend time with.

- **Set Personal Boundaries:** Assertively communicate your boundaries and preferences to others. Do not hesitate to say no or remove yourself from uncomfortable situations.

- **Digital Safety:** Be mindful of what you share on social media and who can access your personal information. Adjust privacy settings to ensure your online presence is secure.

- **Self-Defense Training:** Consider enrolling in a self-defense class or workshop to learn physical techniques and gain confidence in protecting yourself. These skills can empower you to respond effectively in threatening situations.

By implementing these strategies and maintaining a proactive mindset, you can enhance your safety while socializing and partying on college or university campuses. Remember, your well-being is paramount, and taking steps to safeguard it is an important part of your college experience.

***

Interacting with Strangers and Acquaintances

Let's discuss the topic of interacting with strangers and acquaintances, focusing on essential strategies to ensure your safety while on college or university campuses. Understanding how to navigate these interactions is crucial for maintaining personal security.

One of the most effective ways to enhance your safety is by developing situational awareness. **Always be mindful of your surroundings**, whether you are walking alone on campus or attending a social event. Trust your instincts and be cautious when encountering unfamiliar individuals. Remember, it is okay to say no or decline invitations that make you feel uncomfortable.

When interacting with strangers, **establish clear boundaries and communicate assertively**. Be cautious when sharing personal information, such as your address or phone number, and avoid disclosing too much too soon. Utilizing technology, such as location-sharing apps, can provide an extra layer of security when meeting someone new.

Building a **network of trusted friends and acquaintances** is also crucial. Surrounding yourself with supportive individuals who share similar safety concerns can help create a safer campus environment. Establishing a buddy system, where you and a friend look out for each other, can be invaluable when attending parties or walking alone at night.

Additionally, **familiarize yourself with campus security resources and protocols**. Take the time to learn about emergency procedures, such as locating emergency call boxes and understanding the campus escort service. Knowing these resources can provide peace of mind and quick assistance in case of an emergency.

Lastly, **trust your intuition and prioritize self-defense education**. Consider enrolling in a self-defense class specifically designed for women. Learning practical techniques to protect yourself can significantly increase your confidence and personal safety.

By implementing these strategies, you can navigate interactions with strangers and acquaintances while prioritizing your safety on college and university campuses. Remember that your well-being is paramount, and being proactive in safeguarding yourself is essential. Stay alert, communicate assertively, build a support network, and familiarize yourself with campus security resources.

10

Preparing for Emergency Situations and Unexpected Events

Comprehensive Safety Planning

"Safety and emergency preparedness is essential."

— Cindy Hyde-Smith

Creating a Personal Safety Plan

In the bustling environment of higher education, it's vital for women enrolled in a college or university to make their personal safety a top priority. Whether you're a student or a concerned parent, establishing a thorough personal safety plan offers reassurance and equips you or your loved ones with the confidence to navigate campus life. This chapter aims to assist you in crafting robust and effective personal safety tactics.

- **Assessing Potential Risks:** The first step in creating a personal safety plan is to identify potential risks and hazards on campus. This includes understanding the layout of the campus, knowing high-risk areas, and becoming familiar with campus security measures.

- **Utilizing Campus Resources:** Most colleges and universities offer various resources to ensure the safety of their students. They should be able to outline the key resources available, such as emergency phone locations, campus security escorts, and self-defense classes.

- **Building a Support Network:** Cultivating a strong support network is essential for personal safety. Build a support network of trusted friends, roommates, or campus organizations that can offer support during challenging situations.

- **Establishing Safety Routines:** Implementing safety routines can significantly reduce risks and we have already discussed with you the importance of always walking in well-lit areas, avoiding isolated places, and communicating travel plans with someone trusted.

- **Securing Personal Belongings:** Theft is a common concern on college campuses. Here, readers will learn how to protect their personal belongings, including securing dorm rooms, using strong passwords for digital accounts, and keeping valuable items out of sight.

- **Developing Self-Defense Skills:** Basic self-defense skills can enhance your personal safety. Refresh your knowledge by reviewing the previous sections on simple techniques and strategies to help you feel more confident and prepared to protect yourself if necessary.

- **Utilizing Technology:** Technology can be a powerful tool in personal safety. Refresh your knowledge with our already explored various safety apps, emergency alert systems, and other digital tools that can be utilized to enhance personal security.

By following the guidelines provided in this subchapter, women at colleges or universities, as well as concerned parents, can create a personal safety plan tailored to their specific needs and circumstances, empowering them to make informed decisions and prioritize their personal well-being.

***

Responding to Active Shooter Scenarios

In today's world, it is crucial to be prepared for any situation, including the possibility of an active shooter scenario on college or university campuses. Let's explore some essential information on how to respond effectively to such an unimaginable event.

- **Stay Alert and Aware:** The first step in responding to an active shooter scenario is to always remain alert and aware of your surroundings. Pay attention to any signs of suspicious activities or individuals, and trust your instincts. If something feels off, it probably is.

- **Run, Hide, Fight:** In an active shooter situation, it is crucial to remember the three basic options: **run, hide, or fight.** If possible, always attempt to run to a safe location. Leave behind your belongings and help others escape if you can. If running is not an option, find a hiding place that offers cover and concealment. Lock or barricade doors if possible and turn off lights. Finally, as a last resort, be prepared to fight for your life.

- **Communication is Key:** During an active shooter situation, it is crucial to effectively communicate with others. Use texts, calls, or social media platforms to inform friends, family, or authorities about your location, the situation, and any relevant information that can aid in your rescue.

- **Practice Evacuation Drills:** Colleges and universities often conduct emergency drills, including active shooter scenarios. Familiarize yourself with the campus emergency procedures and participate actively in these drills. Knowing the layout of buildings, evacuation routes, and safe locations can significantly increase your chances of survival.

- **Mental and Physical Preparedness:** Being mentally and physically prepared can make a significant difference during an active shooter scenario. Stay updated on self-defense techniques, such as basic strikes and escapes, and consider taking a self-defense class specifically designed for women. Additionally, practice stress management techniques to help maintain a clear mind during high-pressure situations.

Remember, no one ever expects to be caught in an active shooter scenario, but being prepared can save lives. Following these guidelines will equip women on college and university campuses with the knowledge and tools necessary to respond effectively to such a terrifying event. By staying alert, understanding the **run, hide, fight** approach, communicating effectively, practicing evacuation drills, and being mentally and physically prepared, women can enhance their personal safety and increase their chances of survival in an active shooter scenario.

✳✳✳

Handling Medical Emergencies and First Aid Basics

In any environment, accidents and medical emergencies can occur unexpectedly. As women attending college or university, it is crucial to be prepared and equipped with the knowledge and skills to handle such situations. We will explore handling medical emergencies and understanding first aid basics.

When faced with a medical emergency, it is important to remain calm and assess the situation. The first step is to ensure your safety and that of the victim. Call for emergency medical assistance immediately, providing accurate details of the incident and location. If possible, ask someone nearby to help you, and don't hesitate to delegate tasks.

Understanding basic first-aid techniques can make a significant difference in the outcome of an emergency. Consider taking a First-Aid class, which will also cover key areas like CPR (cardiopulmonary resuscitation), which is a life-saving technique used in cases of cardiac arrest. You will learn step-by-step instructions so that you can confidently perform CPR until professional help arrives.

You will also learn how to recognize and respond to common medical emergencies such as severe bleeding, choking, seizures, allergies, and fractures. You will learn how to apply pressure to control bleeding, perform the Heimlich maneuver, assist someone having a seizure, and properly immobilize a suspected fracture.

Furthermore, it is essential to be knowledgeable about the basics of first aid kits and their contents for providing immediate care during minor injuries or medical emergencies. Assemble a well-stocked first aid kit that includes items such as bandages, antiseptics, gloves, and medications for common ailments, and regularly check and replenish the supplies to ensure its readiness in times of need. Here are the basics of first aid kits and their typical contents:

First Aid Kit Essentials:

- **Container:** First aid kits come in various sizes and types, such as plastic boxes, bags, or cases. Choose one that is durable, portable, and water-proof to keep contents protected.

Basic Supplies:

- **Adhesive Bandages:** Various sizes and shapes for minor cuts and wounds.

- **Sterile Gauze Pads or Dressings:** Used to cover wounds or stop bleeding.

- **Medical Tape:** Secures dressings or bandages in place.

- **Antiseptic Wipes or Solution:** For cleaning wounds and preventing infection.

- **Disposable Gloves:** To protect the caregiver from bodily fluids or contamination.

Medications:

- **Pain Relievers:** Over-the-counter pain relievers like acetaminophen or ibuprofen.

- **Antihistamines:** Useful for allergic reactions or insect bites.

Tools and Equipment:

- **Scissors:** Used for cutting bandages or clothing if needed.

- **Tweezers:** For removing splinters or foreign objects.

- **Thermometer:** To monitor body temperature.

- **CPR Mask:** Provides a barrier while performing CPR.

Emergency Information:

- **First Aid Manual:** Offers guidance on basic first aid procedures.

- **Emergency Contact Information:** Include emergency phone numbers and medical history details if relevant.

Additional Items (Depending on Need):

- **Burn Cream or Gel:** For treating minor burns.

- **Eye Wash Solution:** In case of eye irritation or foreign objects in the eye.

- **Instant Cold Packs:** To reduce swelling or relieve pain.

- **Emergency Blanket:** For maintaining body temperature in extreme conditions.

Maintenance Tips:

- **Regular Check-ups:** Periodically inspect and replenish expired or used items.

- **Personalize According to Needs:** Tailor the kit based on specific activities, environments, or family needs.

A well-equipped first aid kit is a fundamental resource for managing minor injuries or providing initial care during emergencies. Regularly maintain and update the kit to ensure it remains fully stocked and ready to use when needed. Understanding the basic contents and their uses can significantly aid in addressing unforeseen medical situations effectively.

Lastly, we want to emphasize the importance of seeking professional medical help and not underestimating the severity of an injury or illness. Familiarize yourself in advance with on-campus health services, nearby hospitals, and emergency contact numbers, ensuring you are aware of the available resources in your college or university.

Being prepared and equipped to handle medical emergencies is an invaluable skill that can potentially save lives.

11

ONLINE SAFETY AND CYBERSECURITY

Safeguard Your Personal Information and Privacy in the Digital Age

Protecting Personal Information and Privacy Online

In this era of digital connectivity, where our lives intertwine more than ever with the virtual realm, women in college or university settings must be knowledgeable about safeguarding personal information and privacy online. We aim to offer valuable insights and practical guidance to navigate the online environment securely and with confidence.

The Internet provides countless opportunities for learning, social interaction, and individual development. Yet it also introduces notable risks like identity theft, cyberbullying, and online harassment. Women, in particular, may face unique challenges and vulnerabilities online. By understanding and implementing effective strategies, they can safeguard their personal information and privacy online.

Above all, it's crucial to be cautious about the information disclosed online. Women should exercise prudence when sharing personal details like full names, addresses, phone numbers, or birthdates on social media platforms or online forums. Overdisclosure can result in unintended outcomes and equip potential wrongdoers with the means to exploit or cause harm.

Ensuring robust and distinctive passwords for every online account is another pivotal facet of safeguarding personal information. Women ought to refrain from employing easily predictable passwords or variations based on their name or birthdate. Employing a mix of uppercase and lowercase letters, numbers, and special characters can notably fortify the security of their accounts.

Additionally, it's crucial to approach unsolicited emails, messages, or friend requests from unfamiliar individuals with skepticism. These could potentially be phishing attempts crafted to deceive women into revealing sensitive information or allowing access to their devices. By exercising caution and confirming the authenticity of such communications, women can avoid becoming prey to malicious schemes.

Consistently adjusting privacy settings on social media platforms and other online accounts is a proactive step to managing the exposure of personal information. By limiting access solely to friends or trusted connections, women can decrease the chances of their data being accessed by unauthorized individuals.

Finally, keeping abreast of present online threats, scams, and privacy issues is paramount. Women should consistently educate themselves on emerging trends and adopt best practices for online safety. This understanding empowers them to make informed choices and implement suitable measures to effectively safeguard their personal information and privacy.

By following these guidelines and adopting a cautious, proactive approach, women can create a secure online environment. The digital world offers endless possibilities, and with the right knowledge and tools, women can navigate it confidently while safeguarding their personal information and privacy.

✳✳✳

Recognizing and Avoiding Online Scams and Threats

Online scams and threats have seen a rise in prevalence. It's vital to comprehend these risks and proactively shield yourself. We'll offer valuable insights and practical advice on identifying and evading online scams and threats, so you can prioritize your digital safety and security.

The Internet offers incredible opportunities for education, communication, and entertainment. However, it also harbors individuals with malicious intentions who seek to exploit unsuspecting victims. From phishing emails to fake social media profiles, online scammers use various tactics to trick individuals into sharing personal information or engaging in fraudulent activities.

To protect yourself from online scams and threats:

- **Be cautious** of unsolicited emails, messages from unknown sources, or offers that seem too good to be true. It is essential to remember that reputable organizations will never ask for sensitive information, such as social security numbers or passwords, through email or instant messaging.

- **Be aware** of online predators. These individuals often masquerade as friendly acquaintances or potential romantic partners, gaining trust before exploiting their victims emotionally or financially. Women should exercise caution when interacting with individuals they meet online and avoid sharing personal details or engaging in intimate conversations until they have established a genuine connection and verified the person's identity.

- **Secure** personal devices and accounts. Women should regularly update their passwords, enable two-factor authentication, and be cautious when connecting to public Wi-Fi networks. It is also advisable to use reputable antivirus software and keep devices up-to-date with the latest security patches.

- **Educate yourself** about the latest online scams and threats. Stay informed by following reliable sources of information, such as cybersecurity blogs or official campus security updates.

- **Take advantage** of the resources and workshops on online safety offered by your college or university to enhance your knowledge and awareness.

By recognizing and avoiding online scams and threats, you can protect yourself from falling victim to cybercriminals. Being proactive, skeptical, and informed is the first step towards maintaining a safe and secure online presence while pursuing your educational goals.

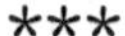

***

Dealing with Cyberbullying and Online Harassment

In today's digital age, where social media and online platforms dominate our lives, cyberbullying and online harassment have become unfortunate realities. Women need to be aware of these issues and equipped with strategies to deal with them effectively. This subchapter will provide guidance and practical advice on how to navigate the digital landscape safely.

The digital world offers numerous benefits, but it also exposes individuals to potential dangers. Cyberbullying and online harassment encompass various forms of mistreatment and hostility conducted through digital platforms and can have severe emotional and psychological consequences. It is essential to recognize the signs and take action promptly. These can include:

Different Forms:

- **Harassment:** Repeated offensive, abusive, or threatening messages directed at an individual, often intended to intimidate or cause distress.

- **Trolling:** Deliberate provocation or incitement of arguments, insults, or offensive comments online.

- **Doxing:** Sharing private or sensitive information about an individual without their consent, leading to invasion of privacy and potential harm.

- **Impersonation:** Creating fake accounts or pretending to be someone else to deceive, manipulate, or harm a person's reputation.

- **Exclusion or Cyberstalking:** Systematically excluding someone from online groups or activities, or persistent, unwanted surveillance and tracking online.

Impact on Mental Health and Well-being:

- **Emotional Distress:** Constant exposure to negative or hurtful content can lead to anxiety, depression, and increased stress levels.

- **Isolation:** Victims may withdraw from social interactions, feeling isolated or disconnected.

- **Low Self-Esteem:** Ongoing harassment can damage self-worth and confidence.

- **Physical Symptoms:** Stress-related physical symptoms like headaches, sleep disturbances, and digestive issues might arise.

Strategies to Cope:

- **Seek Support:** Reach out to friends, family, or counselors for emotional support.

- **Document and Report:** Save evidence of harassment and report it to the platform or authorities.

- **Limit Exposure:** Minimize interactions with the perpetrator and block or mute them where possible.

- **Self-care:** Prioritize activities that promote relaxation and well-being.

Prevention:

- **Educate and Raise Awareness:** Spread awareness about the impact of cyberbullying and promote respectful online behavior.

- **Empowerment:** Encourage individuals to stand up against online harassment and support victims.

- **Strict Policies:** Advocate for platforms and organizations to implement strict policies against cyberbullying and harassment.

Dealing with cyberbullying and online harassment requires effective strategies. Here are practical tips to protect personal information, maintain privacy settings, and report abusive behavior on various platforms:

Protecting Personal Information:

- **Limit Information Sharing:** Be cautious about disclosing personal details like addresses, phone numbers, or birthdates on public platforms.

- **Customize Privacy Settings:** Regularly review and adjust privacy settings on social media to control who can view personal information or posts.

- **Strong Passwords:** Employ strong, unique passwords for each account to prevent unauthorized access.

Maintaining Privacy Settings:

- **Platform Settings Review:** Explore privacy settings on social media platforms and customize them according to personal comfort levels.

- **Control Audience:** Adjust who can view posts, profiles, or contact information within platform settings.

- **Limit Location Sharing:** Avoid sharing exact locations or consider using settings that only share general location information.

Reporting Abusive Behavior:

- **Platform Reporting Tools**: Utilize reporting features available on platforms to flag abusive content or behavior.

- **Document Evidence**: Keep records or screenshots of offensive content or interactions as evidence when reporting.

- **Seek Platform Support**: Reach out to platform support or community guidelines for guidance on reporting harassment.

Responding to Cyberbullying and Harassment:

- **Don't Engage:** Avoid retaliating or engaging in arguments; it may escalate the situation.

- **Block and Mute:** Block or mute individuals involved in harassment to minimize exposure to their content.

- **Seek Support:** Talk to trusted friends, family, or counselors for emotional support and guidance.

Additional Tips:

- **Stay Informed:** Regularly update yourself on privacy settings and security features available on different platforms.

- **Educate Others:** Share information about online safety and respectful behavior with peers and community members.

- **Report to Authorities:** If harassment escalates or becomes threatening, report it to law enforcement.

Moreover, resources and support systems are available on college and university campuses, such as counseling services and online reporting systems. Implementing these strategies, such as protecting personal information, managing privacy settings, and promptly reporting abusive behavior, can help individuals mitigate the impact of cyberbullying and online harassment. Staying vigilant and informed while employing these measures promotes a safer and more secure online experience. We also want to emphasize the significance of fostering a supportive and inclusive online community and encourage women to intervene when witnessing cyberbullying or online harassment and to stand up against such behavior. Becoming an active bystander can help create a safer digital environment for all.

Lastly, the role of parents in supporting their daughters through cyberbullying and online harassment incidents is vital. We encourage parents to open up conversations about online safety and maintain open lines of communication with their children. Parents can always recognize the signs of distress in their children better than anyone else can, and will know how to offer support in a helpful and non-judgmental manner.

By equipping you with the necessary knowledge and strategies, this subchapter aims to empower you to navigate the digital world confidently, ensuring your safety and well-being.

12

CREATING A SAFETY CULTURE ON CAMPUS

Active Engagement in Promoting a Safe Campus Environment

"Your own safety is at stake when your neighbor's wall is ablaze."

— Horace

Promoting Bystander Intervention and Active Engagement

In recent years, the importance of promoting bystander intervention and active engagement in creating safer college and university campuses has gained significant recognition. This subchapter will highlight the significance of their role in promoting a culture of safety.

Bystander intervention refers to the act of stepping in or taking action when witnessing a potentially dangerous situation or act of violence. It recognizes that everyone has a responsibility to look out for one another and create a community that is intolerant of violence. By educating women about the power they possess as bystanders, we can foster an environment where they feel comfortable and confident in taking action.

Let's begin by emphasizing the importance of being an active bystander and the positive impact it can have on campus safety. We will explore various strategies and techniques that women can use to intervene safely and effectively, such as speaking up, seeking help from authorities, and offering support to potential victims in ways that minimize harm and maximize their own safety. Being an active bystander involves safely and effectively intervening in situations where someone might be at risk or facing harm. Here are various strategies and techniques that women, or anyone, can utilize to intervene as active bystanders:

Direct Approaches:

- **Distract or Interrupt:** Intervene by creating a distraction or interrupting the situation to de-escalate tension.

- **Engage in Conversation:** Approach the individuals involved and initiate a conversation to diffuse the situation calmly.

- **Ask for Help:** Involve others nearby by seeking their assistance or calling for help together.

Delegate Actions:

- **Alert Authorities:** Contact security personnel, law enforcement, or emergency services if the situation is escalating or potentially dangerous.

- **Find a Responsible Party:** Locate someone in authority or a person responsible for handling such situations and seek their intervention.

Support the Targeted Person:

- **Offer Support:** Approach the individual being targeted and express concern or offer assistance to remove them from the situation.

- **Create Distraction for Exit:** Provide an opportunity for the targeted person to safely exit by creating a diversion or inviting them to another location.

Create a Distraction:

- **Make Noise:** Attract attention by making noise or calling out for help to gather bystanders and deter the aggressor.

- **Use a Distraction:** Drop something, make a loud sound, or create a diversion to redirect attention from the situation.

Promote a Safe Environment:

- **Discuss Boundaries:** Encourage and maintain an atmosphere where respect and boundaries are valued and discussed openly.

- **Educate Others:** Spread awareness about the importance of active bystander intervention and its role in preventing harmful situations.

Safety Precautions:

- **Assess the Situation:** Prioritize personal safety and assess the risks before intervening. Avoid endangering yourself in the process.

- **Involve Others:** If possible, involve other bystanders to ensure collective support and a safer intervention.

Being an active bystander involves employing various strategies to intervene safely and effectively. It's essential to assess the situation, prioritize personal safety, and choose the most suitable approach to de-escalate or prevent harm while promoting a safe and supportive environment for everyone involved. Active engagement can help to promote a safe campus environment. We encourage women to actively participate in campus safety programs, workshops, and community initiatives. By engaging in these activities, women can not only enhance their personal safety skills but also contribute to the overall safety and well-being of the campus community.

For parents of women away at colleges or universities, this subchapter serves as a guide for understanding the role they can play in promoting bystander intervention and active engagement. It provides parents with insight into the importance of open communication with their daughters about campus safety, raising awareness about potential risks, and empowering them to be vigilant and proactive.

Overall, this subchapter seeks to inspire women at colleges or universities and their parents to become catalysts for change. By promoting bystander intervention and active engagement, we can create a campus environment where everyone feels safe, supported, and empowered to take action against violence.

✳✳✳

Creating Safe Spaces and Support Networks

In today's society, women face unique challenges when it comes to their safety, especially on college and university campuses. We're here to empower women by providing them with essential knowledge and practical strategies to navigate these challenges. In this subchapter, we will delve into the importance of creating safe spaces and support networks for women on campus.

One of the key aspects of ensuring women's safety on college campuses is the establishment of safe spaces. These are physical locations where women can feel secure, supported, and free from harassment or harm. Educational institutions must implement policies and procedures that facilitate the creation and maintenance of these safe spaces. This can include enhanced lighting, security cameras, and emergency call boxes, as well as designated women-only areas where women can study, relax, or seek refuge.

However, safety is not solely the responsibility of the institutions; it is a collective effort. Women must come together and form support networks that provide emotional, mental, and physical assistance. Build strong support networks by fostering connections with like-minded individuals and organizations on campus. We emphasize the importance of joining women's clubs, attending workshops, and participating in self-defense classes. These activities not only enhance personal safety but also promote a sense of community, solidarity, and empowerment.

We want to also highlight the significance of open and honest communication between parents and their daughters, allowing for a mutual understanding of safety concerns and the exchange of ideas on how to address them effectively. We have also offered guidance on assisting women in finding and utilizing campus resources, such as counseling services and reporting mechanisms for incidents of violence or harassment.

Creating safe spaces and support networks is not just about physical safety; it is about fostering an environment where women can thrive academically, socially, and emotionally, so they can navigate their college years with confidence, resilience, and a strong support system. By taking an active role in their safety, women will undoubtedly contribute to a safer and more inclusive campus experience for all.

***

Advocating for Policy Changes and Campus Safety Initiatives

In recent years, the issue of campus safety has gained significant attention, and for good reason. Women at colleges or universities, as well as their concerned parents, are increasingly aware of the need for adequate safety measures and policies that protect their well-being. This subchapter aims to empower women and their families with the knowledge and tools necessary to advocate for policy changes and campus safety initiatives.

When it comes to safety on college and university campuses, it is crucial to understand that individual actions alone cannot solve the problem. While personal safety and self-defense strategies are important, they should be complemented by comprehensive institutional policies that prioritize the welfare of students.

One of the first steps in advocating for policy changes is to raise awareness about the issue. Sharing personal experiences or stories from other women can be a powerful tool in highlighting the need for change. By bringing these concerns to the attention of the wider community, women and their supporters can stimulate conversations and encourage action.

Furthermore, it is essential to form alliances with like-minded individuals and organizations on campus. Joining forces with student groups, women's organizations, or campus safety committees can amplify your voice and increase the chances of implementing meaningful changes. Together, you can brainstorm ideas, develop strategies, and create a united front when advocating for improvements in campus safety.

When engaging with campus authorities or policymakers, it is important to approach them with well-researched proposals by conducting research, collecting data, and understanding the legal framework surrounding campus safety. By presenting evidence-based arguments and concrete solutions, women and their allies can make compelling cases for policy changes that address their concerns.

In addition to advocating for policy changes, we emphasize the importance of supporting existing campus safety initiatives. Explores various initiatives such as self-defense classes, campus escort services, and emergency response systems. By actively participating in these programs, women can not only enhance their personal safety but also demonstrate their commitment to a safer campus environment.

Remember, change takes time and persistence. By advocating for policy changes and campus safety initiatives, women can contribute to a safer future for all. Together, let us work towards creating an environment where women, and all students alike, can pursue their education without fear or compromise.

13

WOMEN'S CAMPUS SAFETY RESOURCE AND SUPPORT SERVICES

An Overview of Campus and Supplemental Safety Resources

Campus Resources for Reporting and Seeking Help

As a woman on a college or university campus, it is essential to be aware of the resources available to you should you ever need to report an incident or seek help. We will provide an overview of the campus resources that can assist you in maintaining your safety and addressing any concerns.

One crucial resource on campus is the campus security or police department. They are responsible for maintaining a safe environment and can be reached in case of emergencies or any suspicious activities. Make sure to have their contact information easily accessible, whether it's programmed into your phone or printed out and kept in your wallet or backpack.

In addition to campus security, most colleges and universities have a dedicated office for Title IX or gender-based violence. These offices are specifically designed to handle reports of sexual misconduct, harassment, or domestic violence. They provide support, guidance, and resources for survivors, as well as educate the campus community on prevention and awareness.

Counseling centers or mental health services are another valuable resource available to you. They offer confidential support for a wide range of issues, including stress, anxiety, depression, and trauma. If you ever feel overwhelmed or need someone to talk to, don't hesitate to reach out to these professionals, who are trained to help.

Furthermore, it is essential to familiarize yourself with the various student organizations and clubs on campus that focus on women's safety, empowerment, or self-defense. These groups often organize workshops, seminars, or self-defense classes specifically tailored to women. Participating in these activities can not only enhance your personal safety skills but also create a supportive network of like-minded individuals.

Lastly, don't underestimate the power of your fellow students. Peer support can be invaluable during challenging times. Establishing connections with your classmates and roommates can provide an additional layer of safety and create a sense of community.

Parents should also be aware of these resources. Encourage your daughters to familiarize themselves with campus safety measures and to reach out for help when needed. Stay informed about any updates or changes to campus safety policies and encourage open communication regarding any concerns or incidents that may arise.

Remember, your safety is a top priority, and utilizing these campus resources can make a significant difference in maintaining a secure and supportive environment for all students on campus.

***

Local and National Organizations Supporting Women's Safety

In recent years, the issue of women's safety on college and university campuses has gained significant attention. More and more women are becoming aware of the importance of their personal safety and are seeking resources and support to ensure their well-being. Thankfully, there are several local and national organizations dedicated to empowering and safeguarding women, both on and off campus.

Local organizations play a crucial role in addressing the specific safety concerns of women within their communities. They often collaborate with colleges and universities to provide workshops, seminars, and training sessions on self-defense and personal safety. These organizations aim to equip women with the necessary skills and knowledge to navigate the challenges they may encounter on campus.

One such local organization is the **SafeCampus** initiative, which partners with universities across the country to create safer environments for students. SafeCampus offers a range of services, including a 24/7 helpline, safety escorts, and educational programs focused on prevention and awareness. By fostering a culture of safety and support, SafeCampus empowers women to take control of their personal security while pursuing their education.

On a national level, organizations like the **National Organization for Women** (NOW) and the **National Women's Law Center** (NWLC) advocate for women's safety and rights. These organizations work tirelessly to address systemic issues that contribute to gender-based violence and discrimination. They engage in policy advocacy, research, and public awareness campaigns to promote gender equality and combat violence against women.

Parents of women attending college or university can also find solace in organizations such as the **Clery Center**. This national organization provides resources and information on campus safety, including the *Jeanne Clery Disclosure of Campus Security Policy* and *Campus Crime Statistics Act*. The Clery Center offers guidance on understanding crime statistics, reporting incidents, and advocating for safer campuses. By arming themselves with knowledge, parents can actively support their daughters in making informed decisions about their safety.

In conclusion, local and national organizations play a pivotal role in supporting and advocating for women's safety on college and university campuses. By collaborating with educational institutions, these organizations empower women with the necessary skills and resources to protect themselves. Furthermore, they work tirelessly to address systemic issues and promote gender equality. Whether through self-defense training, advocacy, or educational programs, these organizations are instrumental in creating safer environments for women pursuing their education. Parents can also find comfort in the resources provided by these organizations, ensuring their daughters' safety remains a priority. Together, we can create a future where women feel safe and empowered to thrive on campus and beyond.

Online Platforms and Apps for Safety and Support

In today's digital age, technology has become an invaluable tool for enhancing women's safety and providing support on college and university campuses. With the rise of online platforms and apps specifically designed to address the unique safety concerns faced by women, it is now easier than ever to access information, resources, and assistance at the touch of a button. This subchapter explores some of the most effective online platforms and apps that can empower women and provide them with a sense of security.

One of the most popular and widely used apps for women's safety is **"Circle of Six."** This app allows users to select six trusted friends or family members as emergency contacts. With just a few taps, users can send an alert to their chosen contacts, informing them of their location and requesting immediate help. Circle of Six also offers information on consent, healthy relationships, and resources for survivors of assault, making it an essential tool for women navigating college and university life.

Another noteworthy platform is **"SafeTrek."** This app ensures that help is just a button press away. By simply holding down a button on the app's interface, users can alert local authorities to their location and dispatch emergency services if necessary. SafeTrek is particularly useful when walking alone at night or in potentially dangerous situations.

For those seeking a comprehensive safety resource, **"Rave Guardian"** is a must-have. This platform offers features such as a virtual safety escort, anonymous tip reporting, and real-time emergency notifications. Rave Guardian also allows users to set a safety timer, which alerts their designated contacts if they fail to check in within a specified timeframe. With its extensive range of tools, Rave Guardian provides women with a powerful safety network right at their fingertips.

In addition to these apps, many college campuses now have their own safety apps and online platforms. These platforms often include features like campus maps, emergency contacts, and safety tips tailored specifically to the campus environment. It is highly recommended that women familiarize themselves with their institution's safety resources and ensure they have the necessary apps installed on their smartphones.

By utilizing these online platforms and apps, women can take proactive measures to enhance their safety and well-being on college and university campuses. Whether it's staying connected with trusted friends, accessing emergency services, or staying informed about campus safety resources, technology has revolutionized the way women can protect themselves. With these tools at their disposal, women can feel more empowered, confident, and secure as they navigate campus life.

14

Conclusion: Empowering Women to Take Charge of Their Safety on Campus

Key Reminders to Ensure Safety First

Recap of Key Takeaways

In this last chapter, we will revisit the important lessons and key takeaways from "The Campus Guardian: A Safety and Self-Protection Handbook for Women in College and University Settings." Whether you are a woman attending a college or university or a concerned parent of a young woman away at school, these key points will serve as a reminder and reference to ensure safety first.

- **Awareness is the first line of defense**: Being aware of your surroundings at all times is crucial. Stay vigilant and trust your instincts. Avoid isolated areas, especially at night, and always have a plan in mind.

- **Establish personal boundaries**: Set clear boundaries and communicate them assertively. Make it known that you deserve respect and expect others to respect your personal space and autonomy.

- **Develop strong communication skills**: Effective communication can diffuse potentially dangerous situations. Learn to assertively say no and express yourself confidently. Practice active listening and be aware of non-verbal cues.

- **Utilize safety resources:** Familiarize yourself with the safety resources available on campus. Know the locations of emergency call boxes, campus security offices, and well-lit pathways. Save important numbers, such as campus security and local law enforcement, in your phone.

- **Travel in groups:** Whenever possible, travel with a trusted friend or in a group, especially during late or early hours. There is strength in numbers, and potential attackers are less likely to target a group of people.

- **Self-defense techniques:** Learn basic self-defense techniques to boost your confidence and empower yourself. Attend self-defense workshops or classes offered on campus or in your community. Practice physical techniques, such as strikes, kicks, and escapes, to effectively protect yourself if needed.

- **Utilize technology for safety:** Take advantage of safety apps and features on your smartphone. Share your location with trusted friends or family members, and use apps that allow you to send distress signals in emergency situations.

- **Be cautious with social media:** Be mindful of the information you share on social media platforms. Avoid disclosing personal details that could compromise your safety or reveal your whereabouts.

- **Trust your instincts:** Your intuition is a powerful tool. If a situation feels unsafe or uncomfortable, trust your gut feelings and remove yourself from the situation.

- **Continue learning and advocating for safety:** Safety is an ongoing process. Stay informed about campus safety policies and initiatives. Advocate for improved safety measures on your campus and encourage open discussions about women's safety.

By remembering and implementing these key takeaways, women on college and university campuses can enhance their personal safety and feel empowered in their daily lives. Parents can also use this information as a guide to support and educate their daughters about staying safe while away at school. Remember, your safety matters, and it is important to take proactive steps to protect yourself and those around you.

***

Encouragement to Implement the Strategies and Techniques

In this subchapter, we would like to extend our encouragement to all the women at colleges or universities, as well as the parents of women away at colleges or universities, to actively implement the strategies and techniques discussed in this handbook. By doing so, you are taking a powerful step towards enhancing your safety and well-being on campus.

We understand that adjusting to college life can be overwhelming, especially for those living away from home for the first time. However, it is crucial to prioritize your safety and be prepared for any potential risks or dangers that may arise. This handbook serves as a comprehensive guide, equipping you with the necessary knowledge and skills to navigate these challenges confidently.

Implementing the strategies and techniques outlined here is not just a recommendation; it is a vital part of your personal security. By being proactive, you will develop a strong sense of empowerment and increase your ability to protect yourself in various situations.

Remember, prevention is key. Take the time to familiarize yourself with your campus, including its layout, security measures, and emergency resources. This will allow you to identify potential risks and plan your daily routine accordingly. By being aware of your surroundings and implementing simple yet effective strategies, you can significantly reduce the likelihood of becoming a target.

Additionally, we strongly encourage you to attend self-defense classes or workshops offered on campus or in the community. These programs provide hands-on training, teaching you practical techniques to defend yourself in case of an attack. By investing your time in learning self-defense, you are equipping yourself with invaluable skills that can potentially save your life.

To the parents reading this handbook, we urge you to support your daughters in their journey towards personal safety. Encourage them to take a proactive approach and implement the strategies outlined here. By discussing these topics openly and providing guidance, you are empowering your daughters to navigate the challenges they may face on campus confidently.

In conclusion, we cannot stress enough the importance of implementing the strategies and techniques discussed in this handbook. By taking an active role in your personal safety, you are reclaiming control over your environment and ensuring a secure college experience. Remember, you have the right to feel safe and empowered on campus, and by embracing these strategies, you are taking a significant step toward achieving that goal.

***

Inspiring Women to Advocate for a Safer Campus Environment

In recent years, there has been a growing concern regarding the safety of women on college and university campuses. Incidents of sexual assault, harassment, and violence have sparked a nationwide conversation, prompting women to take charge of their own safety. This subchapter aims to inspire women to become advocates for a safer campus environment, empowering them to make a difference and create positive change.

For women at colleges or universities, it is crucial to be aware of the risks and challenges they may face. By understanding the importance of personal safety and self-defense, women can take proactive measures to protect themselves and support their peers. We emphasize the need for women to come together to form alliances with organizations that work towards creating a safer campus environment.

One of the most effective ways to advocate for change is by raising awareness. Women should be encouraged to organize workshops, panel discussions, and awareness campaigns to educate their fellow students, faculty, and administrators about the issues surrounding women's safety on campus. By sharing personal experiences and highlighting statistics, they can shed light on the gravity of the situation and garner support from the community.

Another essential aspect of advocacy is collaborating with campus security and administration. Women should be encouraged to establish relationships with campus police, security personnel, and administrative staff. By working closely with these individuals, women can voice their concerns, suggest improvements, and actively participate in the decision-making processes related to safety measures on campus.

Parents also play a significant role in advocating for a safer campus environment. Address your daughters' concerns and support them by staying informed about the safety policies and resources available on campus, while also encouraging open conversations about their personal safety and self-defense.

Furthermore, we also emphasize the importance of self-care and supporting survivors of sexual assault or violence. Women should be encouraged to create safe spaces where survivors can share their stories, seek support, and find healing. By fostering a compassionate and inclusive community, women can create an environment that encourages survivors to come forward and seek justice.

In conclusion, inspiring women to advocate for a safer campus environment is a crucial step toward addressing the issues of women's safety on college and university campuses. By raising awareness, collaborating with campus security and administration, involving parents, and supporting survivors, women can create positive change and ensure a safer future for themselves and their peers.

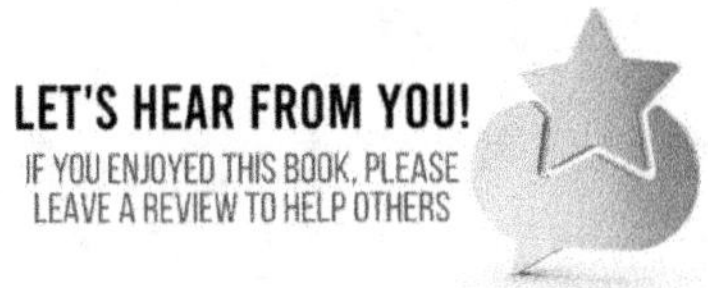

Thank you for reading!